T0344387

Which Treatment Is Best?
Spoof or Proof?

A young woman cries, "Please don't let me die!" Has she received the best treatment? What is the best treatment? How do we know? Life-threatening disease prompts these questions in everyone. *Which Treatment Is Best? Spoof or Proof?* explains the best scientific evidence for any treatment—the randomized controlled trial. This book begins with rotten humor as the source of all diseases. The reader is guided through serious attempts in history to treat disease, but which now seem amusing. The story ends with the randomized controlled trial and how to interpret it. The text will help students and clinicians understand this universal language of clinical research worldwide.

Key Features

- Describes the development of the randomized controlled trial as the gold standard of proof

- Unravels the meaning of "randomized," "double-blind," and "p-values" in a simplified manner for students and clinicians

- Contains timeless information on how medical evidence can be understood

Which Treatment Is Best?
Spoof or Proof?

Teddy Bader, MD

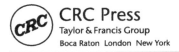
CRC Press
Taylor & Francis Group
Boca Raton London New York

CRC Press is an imprint of the
Taylor & Francis Group, an **informa** business

First edition published 2023
by CRC Press   .
6000 Broken Sound Parkway NW, Suite 300, Boca Raton, FL 33487-2742

and by CRC Press
4 Park Square, Milton Park, Abingdon, Oxon, OX14 4RN

CRC Press is an imprint of Taylor & Francis Group, LLC

© 2023 Teddy Bader

ISBN: 978-1-032-34834-6 (hbk)
ISBN: 978-1-032-34818-6 (pbk)
ISBN: 978-1-003-32405-8 (ebk)

DOI: 10.1201/9781003324058

Typeset in Palatino
by SPi Technologies India Pvt Ltd (Straive)

I wish to dedicate this book to two of my teachers.
Dr. Gene Heasley, at Southern Nazarene University, Oklahoma City,
Oklahoma, taught me how to think about science in general.
And Telfer Reynolds, MD, University of Southern California,
helped me think about the best in clinical therapy years before
the term "evidence-based medicine" was coined.

Contents

Preface

"Doctor don't let me die," sobs a young woman. Her cries penetrate the physician's mind. "Have I given the best medicine? How do I know? What proof is there?"

The book cover illustrates this tension. The teenage sister of German artist Ivo Salinger was diagnosed with acute leukemia in 1918. For two years, Salinger took his sister across the border to Swiss clinics for treatment. She died in 1920. He was so impressed with the care given to her that he painted the picture and gave it to the Swiss physicians who attended her. It depicts a doctor trying to keep the skeleton of death from snatching his patient. The picture has no official title, but my name is, "Physician Struggles with Death."

While there are treatments for everything, the question is do they work? Not only that but are these treatments harmful in subtle ways? Most untested medical therapies are either ineffective or even harmful. The harm is often explained away as a complication of the disease being treated. The presentation here is to help the reader find the gold in treatments proven effective and safe by proper scientific testing.

One would expect the method enabling us to conquer disease and restrain death to be recounted so often that we would tire of the story. Not so. There are only limited accounts of the randomized controlled trial. This text attempts to rectify the situation.

The story describes the humoral medical theory that held sway for more than 2,000 years. Then smallpox vaccination begins an era of comparing numbers. Next, we tell stories of charlatans and testimonials. Later, we focus on controlled trials. Extracts of humor help keep the reader's interest.

Mathematics is kept to a bare necessity. There is no attempt to teach medical statistics. My focus is the randomized controlled trial and the interpretation of the probability value.

I have worked in the trenches. I conceived of a randomized controlled trial, applied for grants to support the substantial expense, took the study to the Food and Drug Administration for a license, and then carried the study to the institutional review board for ethical and operational review. I hired staff, and together we recruited, enrolled, and randomized patients. Trial data was maintained and analyzed. It was submitted to a peer-reviewed publication. It was defended and then published. This was a seven-year stepwise process.

Regarding historical eras, the terms "AD, BC" are used. Professor John Hale, a working archaeologist and academic, states these terms are much less confusing when excavating a site than the similar sounding "CE, BCE" names. AD when written before the date traditionally meant anno domini, whereas now when written after a date, it means "advancing dates"; BC now means "backward count."

Teddy Bader, MD
Professor of Medicine (Retired)
University of Oklahoma Health Sciences Center
Oklahoma City, Oklahoma
tedbader@cox.net

Author

Teddy Bader, MD, is a retired Professor of Medicine from the University of Oklahoma. Dr. Bader worked in the Gastroenterology Section. His effort was centered on liver disease and transplantation. He authored a textbook on viral hepatitis that went into three editions. Dr. Bader penned 55 medical publications that have been cited by 1,131 other scientific reports (Google Scholar). He grew up in Boulder, Colorado. Dr. Bader graduated from Southern Nazarene University in Oklahoma City and Washington University School of Medicine in St. Louis. Married for 49 years to Marilyn, he loves to birdwatch, collect humorous anecdotes, and read history books.

Abbreviations

AIDS	Acquired immunodeficiency syndrome
AMA	American Medical Association
AZT	Zidovudine
BMJ	*British Medical Journal*
FDA	Food and Drug Administration, United States
FRC	Federal Radio Commission
HIV	Human immunodeficiency virus
NEJM	*New England Journal of Medicine*
NIH	National Institutes Health, United States
PAS	Para-aminosalicylic acid
RCT	Randomized control trial
TB	Tuberculosis
WDHW	Transliteration of Ancient Egyptian writing meaning "rotten stuff"
WHO	World Health Organization

1 Early Egyptian Medicine

Egypt, 1500 BC. The New Kingdom reaches peak prosperity in a civilization that will last three millennia. Colossal pyramids have existed for a thousand years. Cleopatra will reign a thousand years later. Papyri are recording medical practices for the first time in world history. Worry about dying and the afterlife influence healing. Given concerns over the afterlife, priests double as religious leaders and physicians.

Death was a constant threat since the average Egyptian lived 30–40 years (98% of modern Americans reach their 40th birthday). While the Nile dwellers feared death, their belief in life after death tempered their apprehension. Knowledge of Egyptian medicine springs from a few surviving manuscripts; adding them together, they would form only a small volume. Egyptians recorded precious little about their civilization. Nothing yet discovered records their description of mummification. Nor do we know the rules of pharaonic succession. Yet, they recorded their ideas of medicine and their prescriptions, though the precise understanding of the ingredients remains speculative. Few Egyptians could read or write. The fact that the priests could do both was essential in their medical leadership.

Medical therapy involved incantations and more rational recipes. Magical spells treated illness. Magic here is defined as a charm or spell that will break the power of sickness. The *Chester Beatty V Papyrus* contains typical spells for healing. One for exorcising a headache begins by asking 20 gods "to remove that enemy which is in the face of N [the patient's name]." The healer must recite the spell "over a crocodile of clay with grain in its mouth." Finally, the spell is to be recited over images of 11 gods "and an Oryx [a type of antelope] on whose back stands a figure [probably the god Horus] carrying a lance."[1]

Amulets were charms to ward off disease-producing demons, while talismans carried positive forces. An amulet manufactured by the thousands in Ancient Egypt shows the eye of the falcon god, Horus. It may have been believed to protect from eye disease—a major problem from blowing desert sand.

The interest in entering the afterlife led to the prohibition of anatomic dissection of cadavers—a sanction common throughout world history until recently. No mutilated person could enjoy the blissful life of the future world. Embalmers were a lower social class separated from contact with the physician priests. Only rich people could afford to be mummified. Mummification was an effort to keep a person whole after death. The embalmers appeared to have acquired little practical anatomy. In any case, knowledge of body structure was not shared between the embalmers and the healers.

Unable to dissect cadavers, Egyptian healers constructed fanciful theories about the function of the body. Most of what we know about Egyptian body function comes from the *Ebers Papyrus* (1550 BC).

THE CHANNELS OF LIFE: METU

Nile dwellers regarded air as vital to life. They imagined air entered the body through the nose and traveled through the trachea directly into the heart. Air left the heart in the blood, along with water, and traveled via a series of outgoing ducts called metu to each of the body's organs (Figure 1.1). From some of the secondary organs, a second set of metu carried those respective products to the surface (e.g., nose produces mucus, bladder urine, testes semen). The healers could not differentiate between arteries, veins, nerves, and tendons, and lumped these all together as metu.[2]

DOI: 10.1201/9781003324058-1

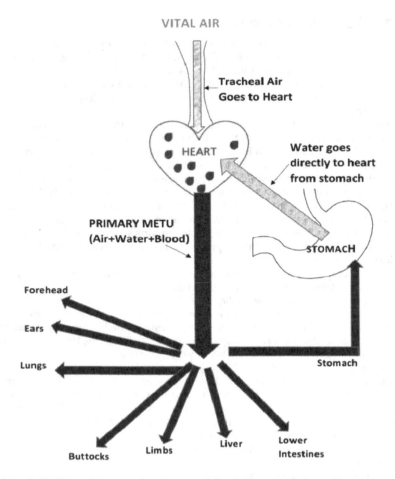

Figure 1.1 Egyptian metu movement of fluid. The stomach and heart were considered in close contact and function. Circulation of body substances should not be implied here. The surging and receding of the Nile River may be a metaphor closer to Egyptian thinking (drawing by author; information collated from Estes).[2]

The importance of metu even to nonphysicians was implicit in everyday ancient wishes, such as "may his metu be comfortable," and in greetings, "may thy metu be sound."[1]

DISORDERED METU

Disordered substance within the metu has been transliterated as "WHDW" (pronounced as "ukhedu") or roughly, in English, "the rotten stuff."[3] As decay and foul odor characterize death, so are they associated with the feces of the living. Upon death, the first organ to deteriorate is the colon or large intestine. WHDW thus originated in the feces. If the WHDW could accumulate to a dangerous level in the rectum, the pathogenic WHDW would overflow into its returning metu and travel backward to the heart. Disease would then be distributed throughout the body. WHDW was surmised to be converted into pus after it entered the metu, and when it settled in an organ, sickness began.

Egyptians used the term, "blood-eater," to describe the WHDW's ability to change the blood and cause disease. Among the terrifying demons in the Hall of Judgment before which a deceased Egyptian had to appear were a "Blood-Eater" and an "Eater-of-Intestines"—both of whom represented fears of corporeal corruption.

Bad blood was detected by its odor. One priest-healer is portrayed as smelling the blood of a sacrificed bull and pronouncing "it is pure." Presumably, this meant there was no WHDW.[4]

RESISTING CORRUPTION

Corruption of the body could be resisted with cleanliness and circumcision. Cleanliness was an everyday concern, even a preoccupation, of Egyptians of all classes. Bathing areas, in which water was poured over the bather while they stood on a stone slab with raised edges, have been found both in private and royal homes. Because hair attracted dirt, beards and body hair were regularly removed, especially by priests, who shaved their heads.

The beard of the Pharaoh was a symbol of authority, but one placed on his chin prior to public appearances. If one looks closely at statues of the Egyptian leaders, indentations of the cheeks betray the straps holding the beards on.

Circumcision, the removal of the penile foreskin, was first practiced in Egypt. The circumcision scene in the Old Kingdom (2300 BC) mastaba (tomb) at Sakkara is the oldest surviving portrayal of any surgical procedure (Figure 1.2).

The putrefying WHDW was also resisted through cathartics and wound ointments. Laxatives formed the principal part of the Egyptian healer's armamentarium to promote health and ward off disease. All classes of the Nile population appear obsessed with keeping the intestines free of the dangerous WHDW. To accomplish this goal, Egyptians regularly took laxatives, so unhealthy amounts of WHDW could not accumulate. This prophylactic habit was so widespread that in the fifth century BC, Herodotus, the Greek traveler and historian, noted with amazement, "they purge themselves every month, three days successively, seeking to preserve health by emetics and clysters [enemas]…and indeed, the Egyptians, next to the Libyans, are the healthiest people in the world."

The Egyptian pharmacopeia contains many cathartics. Nile dwellers were the first to use castor oil in this role, a use that survives into twenty-first-century America. Even today, traces of the WHDW can be detected in televised advertisements that urge us to use laxatives to improve our outlook on life and interpersonal relationships.

Wound ointments were the second major product healers prescribed. The most frequent ingredient in ancient Nile medicines was honey. Dr. Estes, a modern physician, has demonstrated in the laboratory the bacteria-inhibiting aspects of honey against *Staphylococcus aureus*, one of the most common causes of severe wound infection.[5]

On the other hand, harm was likely to ensue from the following prescription—"use the fresh dung of an ass, heated and bound with a cloth, and place it on the sore eyes."[6]

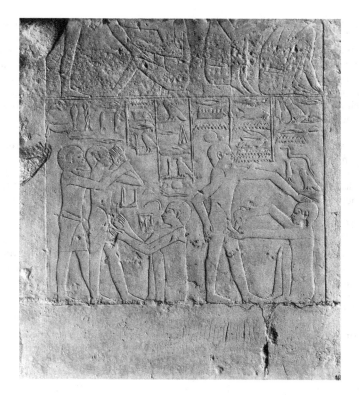

Figure 1.2 Sakkara, Egypt. Wall carving of circumcision scene. In the right-hand panel, the priest appears to be making the incision with a flint blade. The pubertal boy says in the panel above him, "Obliterate real thoroughly!" and the operator replies, "I will make it agreeable!" An adjacent second priest and patient panel shows the priest applying a post-operative dressing to a restrained patient, and the inscription above says, "Hold him fast!" and "Don't let him swoon." This is the oldest illustration of any surgical procedure in the world. (Circa 2300 BC. From Wellcome Library, London under CC-BY 4.0.)

A PERFUMED PRESCRIPTION

The use of birth control and abortion were severely punished. The Egyptians had a curious notion about the uterus, in that it was subject to frequent fits of wandering about in the pelvic cavity. A woman suffering from a uterine disorder stood over hot coal, on which scented wax was sprinkled. The perfumed smoke rising to the genitalia was then expected to lure the errant uterus back to its normal place. This practice, known as "fumigation," was picked up by the Greeks and Romans and remained a time-honored treatment for uterine disorders until the nineteenth century.

THE LONG-LASTING THEORIES OF EGYPT

What were the contributions of Ancient Egyptians to medicine? Amulets and talismans to ward off disease exist today. It is likely we would have these charms, whether or not the Egyptians owned them. The anxiety of illness leads to a desire for a magical outcome.

The practice of male circumcision continues, and perfume fumigation for female disorders was abandoned only a century ago. Corporal corruption came from the WHDW. Laxatives purged the WHDW. The cleansing of the WHDW remained the center of medical therapeutics until the late nineteenth century.

NOTES

1 Estes JW. *The Medical Skills of Ancient Egypt*. New York: Science History Publications/USA; 1993, p. 7.

2 Ibid, pp. 79–84.

3 Da Silva Veiga PA. *Health and Medicine in Ancient Egypt: Magic and Science: Archaeopress*; 2009, p. 46. DOI: 10.30861/9781407305004

4 Gordon A. *The Quick and the Dead: Biomedical Theory in Ancient Egypt*. Leiden: Brill; 2004, pp. 173–4.

5 Estes, pp. 68–71.

6 Estes, p. 114.

2 Hippocrates, Galen, and the Humoral Theory

Ancient Greece. 500 to 300 BC. The golden age. Art and sculpture multiply. The Parthenon is constructed. Socrates and Plato teach philosophy. Hippocrates (hip-poc-rat-tees) produces the next body of medical literature on the Aegean island of Cos. While all Ancient Egyptian writings on medicine would fill one modest volume, Hippocrates and his associates wrote the equivalent of more than 20 volumes. Descendants of his approach penned many more and added the name of Hippocrates to lend authority.[1]

Born in 460 BC, Hippocrates was a contemporary of Socrates and Plato. Hippocrates was steered into medicine because his physician father dreamed his son should be a doctor. His father was a disciple of a therapy paradigm that used dream interpretation to guide decisions and treatment.

Dissatisfied with the facilities of his medical school on Cos, Hippocrates visited other principal cities to collect and share ideas. While doing so, his reputation grew to the point where he became the most famous physician of his time. Plato recognized the importance of Hippocratic teaching in medicine.

The image of Hippocrates has survived on ancient coins. These coins show Hippocrates to be bald, with prominent eyes and a beard. The origin of this appearance appears to have come from the time when the Hippocratic collection was assembled at Alexandria in the third century BC.

Hippocrates moved medicine from magic to a rudimentary scientific approach by stressing keen observation of the patient. He took a complete history of the patient's symptoms—before their illness and during the illness. He asked about diet, family illnesses, and personal habits. While this hardly seems revolutionary, previous physicians were more interested in the disease itself. The disease was a separate entity from the patient since it was sent as an affliction by the gods. The reason for the divine visitation consumed the attention of pre-Hippocratic physicians, rather than the condition of the poor, wretched patient. Our terminology reflecting divine visitation persists today, as our word for "stroke" (an acute reduction of blood to the brain causing paralysis) derives from the concept that the gods "strike" a man or woman down. Indeed, as this disease develops over a few minutes, such an interpretation seems common sense. Not so to Hippocrates. He was interested in the association between disease and patient. This connection culminated in a complete examination of the patient. Included in this examination was an inspection of all body secretions. This change in focus emphasized the natural history of disease. If the gods do not cause disease, then it must have a predictable outcome. Hippocrates stressed finding the clues during the patient encounter that foretold recovery or death.

He begins his Book of Prognostics,

> It is impossible to make all the sick well; this, indeed, would be better than to be able to foretell what is going to happen; but since men die...and some die immediately after calling him, having lived only a day or longer, and before the physician could bring his art to counteract the disease. ... A man will be esteemed as a good physician for having long anticipated everything; and by seeing and announcing beforehand those who will live and those who will die, he will thus escape censure.[2]

Indeed, this has been the main contribution of Hippocrates throughout the ages. The ability to prognosticate separates physicians and laymen. That is, a layman can prescribe a treatment for a symptom, but has difficulty ascertaining if it made any difference in the condition. The father of medicine would comment,

DOI: 10.1201/9781003324058-2

"The physician who cannot inform his patient what would be the probable issue of his complaint, if allowed to follow its natural course, is not qualified to prescribe any rational plan of treatment for its cure."[1]

Classical Greek public opinion condemned the dissection of the human body. It is likely, however, that Hippocrates performed limited postmortem examinations. Even so, he did not seem to understand the difference between arteries, veins, ligaments, and nerves; he assumed all to have similar function. As a result, he continued the fanciful anatomy and physiology of the Egyptians.

THE HUMORAL THEORY

Humors were tissue fluids in the body, including blood. The Greeks observed four elements in blood after it clots,

1. A dark clot

2. A red fluid

3. Yellow serum

4. Fibrin

This quartet of findings was satisfactory to the Hippocratic School, as Aristotle postulated the four basic elements of earth as fire, earth, water, and air. Moreover, these four elements each had two essential qualities (Figure 2.1).[3]

The yellow bile, secreted in the liver, represented the hot and dry properties; the black bile, arising from the spleen, had cold and dry characteristics; the phlegm, formed in the brain, the cold-moist quality; and the blood, originating from the heart, the hot-moist quality. The humors varied with the season of the

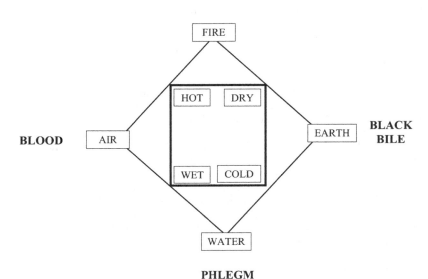

YELLOW BILE

FIRE

HOT   DRY

BLOOD   AIR   EARTH   **BLACK BILE**

WET   COLD

WATER

PHLEGM

Figure 2.1 The relationship, according to Aristotle, between the qualities, the elements, and the humors. (Drawn by author.)

year, the wind, warmth, cold, sunshine, shadow, manner of life, and age. Health depended on the equilibrium and balance of humors. Individuals had their own blend of humors. Disease occurred when proportions became unbalanced.

For example, too much phlegm caused pneumonia. Secreted by the brain, the cold-moist humor dripped down the throat and settled into the lungs. "Proof" came from the observations that lung infections often occur in the cold season of the year and in the "cold constitutions" of the aged.

In the spring, with warm sunshine and rain, there was a predominance of the warm-moist fluid, blood. This mandated that even healthy patients needed a preventative bloodletting in spring, or at least a course of laxatives, to purify the blood.

The humoral theory placed personalities and food into categories. For example, the hot and moist personality was sanguine (i.e., hopeful and positive). The cold and dry temperament was melancholic (depressive or gloomy). Melancholiacs should therefore avoid vegetarian diets (i.e., cold and moist) and eat hot and moist foods, such as meat. Sanguines should eat little meat and more vegetables. Or so the theory of opposites went. The use of opposites was necessary to balance the humors.

Hippocrates divided the course of a disease into three stages. First, an imbalance of body humors was caused by internal or external factors. Second, the body reacted by producing a coction to rebalance the humors that are left in excess.[4] Heat production or fever was one sign of coction. The final phase was a "crisis" with a discharge of excessive humor (via blood, phlegm, vomit, feces, urine, or sweat). A successful crisis led to improvement and a return to health, while an unsuccessful crisis led to death.

Hippocrates remains famous for three statements in modern medicine. "Primum non nocere" (First, do no harm) is the most quoted medical aphorism (either as Latin or English) in the teaching experience of this author. His saying helps offset the strong impetus in acute illness or trauma to "do something," even if the idea is ill-considered or experimental.

Second, "Life is short, the art long, the occasion fleeting, experience fallacious, and judgment difficult."

Third, the Hippocratic Oath is still repeated by many graduating physicians worldwide,

> I swear by Apollo, the physician, Asclepius, and Health, and Panacea, and all the gods and goddesses, that according to my ability and judgment, I will keep this oath and this stipulation: to reckon him who taught me this art equally dear to me as my parents, to share my substance with him, and relieve his necessities if required. … I will give no deadly medicine to anyone if asked, nor suggest any such counsel; and in like manner, I will not give a pessary to produce abortion. With purity and holiness, I will pass my life and practice my Art. I will not cut persons laboring under the stone but will leave this to be done by men who are practitioners of this work. Into whatever houses I enter, I will go into them for the benefit of the sick, and I will abstain from every voluntary act of mischief and corruption, and further, from the seduction of females or males, of freedman or slaves. Whatever, in connection with my professional practice, or not in connection with it, I see or hear, in the life of men, which ought not to be spoken of abroad, I will not divulge as reckoning that all such should be kept secret. While I continue to keep this oath inviolate, may it be granted to me to enjoy life and the practice of the Art, respected by all men, in all times! But should I trespass or violate this oath, may the reverse be my lot![5]

Hippocrates died in Thessaly, but at what age is uncertain. Sources have credited him with a lifetime of 85 to 109 years.

GALEN

Claudius Galenus, commonly known as Galen, was born at Pergamum (now the western coast of Turkey) around 130 AD. His father, Nicon, was a mathematician and lover of Greek literature. At age 14, Galen attended lectures given by many philosophers. Like the father of Hippocrates 600 years earlier, Galen's father was also persuaded by a dream from Apollo that his 17-year-old son should succeed in medicine. In his late teens, Galen became an attendant of the god Asclepius in the temple at Pergamum for four years. After his father's death in 150 AD, Galen traveled to Smyrna (now Izmir, Turkey) to study anatomy. He went to the leading academic center of Alexandria. Their patients from all parts of the world and physicians from every school of philosophy gave him broad exposure to medicine. In 157 AD, he returned to Pergamum, preceded by a reputation, since he had already written treatises on the anatomy and function of the human body. At the age of 28, he was appointed to the prestigious position of doctor to the School of Gladiators (in Pergamum), a charge he held for four years. The injuries suffered by the gladiators provided Galen with further insight into actual human anatomy and allowed him to improve his surgical technique. The daily lives of the gladiators are described in Galen's writings.

Galen traveled to Rome for the first time in AD 163. Introduced to the famous philosopher, Eudemus, Galen cured the thinker of a serious malady that had defied the best efforts of local physicians. Before long, his learning and success earned him the titles of "wonder-speaker" and "wonder-worker." During his time in Rome, he also wrote with the greatest admiration about Hippocrates. Galen claimed to only repeat and further expound the principles of his famous predecessor.

Galen's attempt to purge anti-Hippocratic errors in others, his fame, and vanity brought him the enmity of nearly every Roman physician. Galen accused his colleagues of jealousy and stupid ignorance, calling them "thieves" and "poisoners." He left Rome to return home to Pergamum for a brief period.

Only the appointment as personal physician to the Roman emperor, Marcus Aurelius, induced Galen to return to the Imperial City. He solidified his position at court after curing a disease of the monarch that Galen claimed, "was the most interesting and remarkable case he had ever treated."

Galen provided noteworthy improvements to the understanding of medicine. He was the first in history to identify those tiny, thread-like tissue bundles that ran through the body as nerves, and to differentiate them from blood vessels and ligaments. Cutting the nerves or the spinal cord at distinct levels in animals gave him definite information as to the source of various paralyses. Severing the spinal cord between the third and fourth cervical vertebrae caused respiration to stop; when performed at lower cervical levels, lesser degrees of quadriplegia were produced.

Galen correctly taught that arteries contained blood, while Hippocrates believed arteries contained air. However, Galen's notions of the heart and circulation were sketchy. He was unaware of the rapid movement of blood throughout the body, nor of its considerable volume.

Galen believed pneuma (air, breath), was the fundamental life force (Figure 2.2). Pneuma was taken into the body by breathing. Pneuma took three forms: animal spirit in the brain, vital spirit in the heart, and natural spirit in the liver.

Vital spirit came from the pneuma, which entered through the trachea into the heart. Galen demonstrated blood in the heart but believed it was produced in

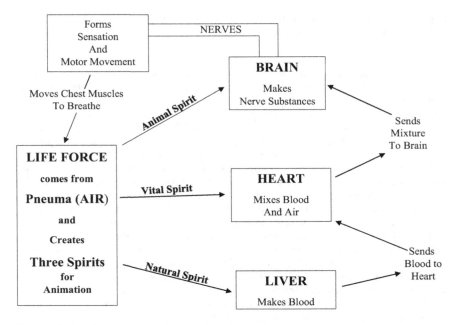

Figure 2.2 Galen's physiology of life force. The life force started at the first breath.

the liver from chyle migrating from the intestines. ("Chyle" is a milky substance taken up from the small intestine during digestion and transported by lymphatic ducts.) The transformation of chyle into blood infused the red fluid with natural spirit. The natural spirit in the liver controlled nutrition, growth, and reproduction.[6]

This activated blood ebbed and flowed through the venous system to the lungs where impurities were removed. The blood passed from the right ventricle to the left ventricle through little pores in the interventricular septum.[7] The blood was thus activated again with the vital spirit. The vital spirit of the heart transported heat and life throughout the body. Reaching the brain, it was activated into the animal spirit and sent through canals in the nerves. Animal spirit generated sensation and movement.

Since human dissection was not permitted in his time, Galen had to content himself with information derived from the dissection of animals. He assumed human organs were the same as lower animals and passed on errors which persisted for centuries. Galen held the human sternum, or breastbone, was divided into sections like the ape; the human uterus had two long horns like a dog, and the hip bone was spread out like an ox.

Galen promoted the idea of "miasma" or foul air. Miasmas could carry the putrefactive particles through the air and cause epidemics of fevers. Fever being literally the disease itself, rather than the symptom of a disease.[8]

Galen is sometimes called the "father of pharmacy" for his fantastic expansion of the list of drugs. Many of his prescriptions are compounded with complicated formulas. Unfortunately, his choices appear to have no rationale for their use beyond the theory of humors. There were cooling remedies in fever, warming drugs for exhaustion, cathartics in constipation, and bloodletting in a plethora (i.e., overabundance of one humor).

There was emphasis on social deportment. The physician should accommodate himself to the patient's habits and level of education. Visits to the bedside should not be made too often. Tactless speeches, such as "Patroclus is dead, and he was a more important man than thou art," were to be avoided.

GALEN'S PRACTICE OF BLOODLETTING

Galen turned bloodletting into a systematic procedure for balancing the humors. There were two approaches. With a small sharply pointed instrument called a lancet, a vein was opened and the patient's venous blood allowed to flow into a basin. This approach was called venesection, phlebotomy, or bloodletting. We will use these latter three terms interchangeably. The most common indication was for the general sign of fever. Second, for an area of local inflammation, the blood was removed from the body part affected. This was called local bloodletting, and it was done by either scarification of the skin from many tiny cuts and then applying a suction cup or by the application of a medicinal leech.

Figure 2.3 illustrates commonly used instruments. The scarificator, developed in the 1600s, used a trigger to send 12 blades into the skin. Cupping glasses were used to draw blood from the skin after scarification. The latter practice was known as wet cupping. In contrast, dry cupping did not use the scarificator. Both cupping approaches involved heating the cup and then placing it on the skin to draw fluid from the tissues.

Medicinal leeches have extracted blood for millennia. *Hirudo medicinalis* is the most common species used. The adult is 20 cm long and uses its anterior sucker to pierce the skin and inject substances that keep the blood from clotting. The leech also injects anesthetic agents. The leech can remove up to 15 mL of blood without harm to the host.

Blood flow was deemed to ebb in a to-and-fro manner, like the tides of the ocean. Given this slow movement, the humoral theory stated bad humors could collect in a body part or area. Thus, it made sense to draw the blood from the area involved.

Galen advocated that the ills of inflammation were so serious that they warranted prophylactic venesection before its expected development, for example, immediately after an injury. The physician from Pergamon used venesection to treat fever, along with cooling drinks. Galen's principal indication, however, was the severity of the patient's disease. The worse the disease, the more blood taken. He was careful to add that the strength of the patient's faculties must be considered, along with his age, previous history, and time of day. These could all be estimated by the strength of the pulse. The pulse was carefully monitored during the operation.

One liter of blood taken away was considered moderate; two liters a heroic removal. More importantly, the removal was to be judged by its effect. In severe illness, evacuation to the point of fainting was vital.

The reader can guess the hazards of bloodletting. Patients with heroic removal would sometimes die suddenly or suffer injury (e.g., blindness).[9] The phlebotomist may have overlooked the fatality from exsanguination (i.e., death from too much blood loss) by attributing the result to the underlying disease or the humoral reasoning of not taking blood soon enough.

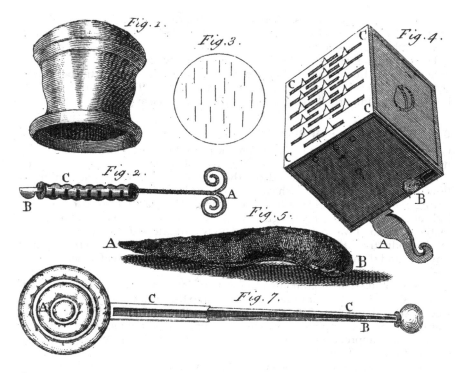

Figure 2.3 Bloodletting instruments, eighteenth century. Fig. 1 is a cup for suction. Fig. 2 is a cutting blade. Fig. 3 shows multiple slits in skin for which a heated cup was placed over to suction blood. Fig. 4 is a scarificator as another way to make skin incisions. Fig. 5 is a leech. Fig. 6 missing. Fig. 7 is a circular lancet with blood drawing chamber. (From Wellcome Library, London, under CC by 4.0.)

GALEN'S LEGACY

Galen died in 201 AD, but his teachings remained the unchallenged authority in medicine for centuries. The reason for this remains speculative for historians. He penned over 500 treatises, large and small, mostly on medical subjects, but also on ethics and logic. His encyclopedic scope and spirit of absolute assurance conveyed an impression of finality, for he asserted he had finished what Hippocrates had begun. Galen's writings comprise more than half of all writings, medical and non-medical, from Ancient Greece!

While Galen was not a Christian, he was a firm monotheist. His platonic demiurge was less personal, however, and comprised a deity who had shaped the material world out of the formless void. Galen looked to the demiurge as an ongoing creative life force. He often repeated Aristotle's dictum, "[N]ature or God never does anything without a purpose." In one book, he praises the love of virtue the Christians possess. These beliefs naturally commended him to the church fathers. But there is more than the support of Christianity to the survival of his system. The Arabs, and subsequently the followers of Mohammed in the seventh century AD, held up his writings as authoritative. These Middle Eastern followers were notable as keepers of many of the manuscripts of Galen for over more than a millennia.

Galen's monotheism made his teachings acceptable to Christians, Jews, and Muslims. As a result, the wisdom of his acknowledged master, Hippocrates, along with the additions made by Galen, reigned over more than the typical limits of Western civilization. The Galenic system of medicine held sway from Persia to North Africa, as well as Europe and the New World. Moreover, it was unchallenged from the third to fifteenth centuries, and many parts of it continued to be practiced well into the twentieth century.

NOTES

1 We will not try to distinguish between Hippocrates and his associates as sources. We will consider Hippocrates and the Hippocratic school as equivalent for our purposes.

2 Adams F. *The Genuine Works of Hippocrates*. London: Sydenham Society; 1849, p. 18.

3 Singer CJ, Underwood EA. *A Short History of Medicine*. London: Oxford University Press; 1962, p. 46.

4 Latin coctio—cooking or digestion.

5 Black, Winston E. *Medicine and Healing in the Premodern West: A History in Documents*. Peterborough, Ontario: Broadview Press; 2020, p. 52, Print.

6 We now understand that the blood is not produced in the liver, but in the bone marrow. Observers were quite uncertain what the function of the liver was until the chemical structure of bile was determined in the nineteenth century. When the liver is freshly removed, it is noted to be the largest solid organ in the body yet appears to only contain a mass of oozing blood and a few drops of bile from its surface. There have been at least 10,000 catalytic chemical reactions reported in the liver so far, and this seems to be a minority of those likely to exist. However, the suppositions of Galen were reasonable given the observable anatomy.

7 These intraventricular pores are rarely seen in humans. Galen's information evidently came from cats and dogs where these connections are common. Again, the reader must not draw the conclusion that Galen's notion of the circulation of blood was cyclical. Rather, the blood moved slowly more like the ebb and tide of the ocean. Most, if not all, of the blood was consumed in the extremities only to have more generated in the liver for the next ocean tide.

8 Steuer R, Saunders J. *Ancient Egyptian and Cnidian Medicine*. Berkeley, CA: University of California Press; 1959, p. 5.

9 Mapleson T. *A Treatise on the Art of Cupping, etc.* London: J. Wilson Publisher (Google Books); 1830, p. 42.

3 Clay Ears and Asclepian Medicine

Few physicians were educated in the classical world. Wealthy aristocrats and the Roman legion recruited the limited number of doctors trained. For everyone else, finding a healer in the classical world was difficult. The poor had limited choices. One possibility was a shrine healing center where medico-religious rituals were performed. Asclepius (pronounced as-clee-pee-us) was the Greek god of healing and medicine. Asclepius was described as in existence no later than the eighth century BC. Coins from the fifth century BC show the face of Asclepius with a beard and a full head of curly hair. His portrait resembles Zeus, but Asclepius's demeanor is kindly rather than stern. Contrary to the nudity of the other gods, he wore a regular male garment known as a himation. The himation was draped over his left shoulder, with his right shoulder exposed. His appearance follows Hippocrates's advice that physicians must be clean and well-dressed.[1]

The cult of Asclepius was widespread in the ancient Mediterranean world from the fourth century BC to the fifth century AD. More than 500 temple sites scattered throughout the Roman Empire were dedicated to the worship of Asclepius.[2]

Asclepius was the son of Apollo. Apollo was one of 12 principal Olympian deities in the Greek and Roman Pantheon. Apollo was the god of healing, poetry, and music. The story of how Asclepius became recognized as the leading god in medicine is convoluted and irrelevant to our history. Asclepius was given the power to heal by Zeus, the chief deity, but was restrained from raising the dead.

THE TEMPLE AT PERGAMUM

One of the notable temples to Asclepius was in Pergamum (on the Mediterranean coast of modern-day Turkey).[3] The temple at Pergamum was founded in 350 BC. In 133 BC, the city of Pergamum demonstrated its own importance by becoming the capital of the Roman province of Asia. Asclepius was at the peak of his celebrity status during the second century AD. Pergamum was also at its greatest size during the second century AD. Moreover, it was the largest Asclepian sanctuary in Asia Minor, as demonstrated by its extensive archaeological remains.

A sacred road, called the Via Tecta, 820 meters long, connected the city and temple in Pergamum (Figure 3.1). The last 40 meters of the road was widened during the reign of Emperor Hadrian to include Corinthian columns flanked by numerous tents of merchants selling sacrifices or votives (small body parts made of gold or clay relating to the presenting physical complaint; Figure 3.2).

A monumental gate separated the sanctuary from the profane entrance. Three types of patients were not allowed into the temple: the acutely ill, the moribund (i.e., near death), and women about to deliver. Reasons for these exclusions are unclear, but the motive may have been to prevent the wails of the dying or the cries of those in labor from disturbing the peace of the sanctuary.

To the north, south, and east, Corinthian columns 10 meters tall surrounded the sanctuary. The portico (a covered walkway) surrounded the complex on three sides. The northern walkway allowed visitors to skirt the sanctuary while moving to the small amphitheater, which could seat about 3,000 people. The performance of comedies or tragedies likely provided psychological help. Other times, the patients participated as a character in a play as part of a therapeutic regimen.

Asclepian temples (Figure 3.3) provided drinking water believed to have special healing properties; water for bathing, ritual cleansing, and hydrotherapy;

DOI: 10.1201/9781003324058-3

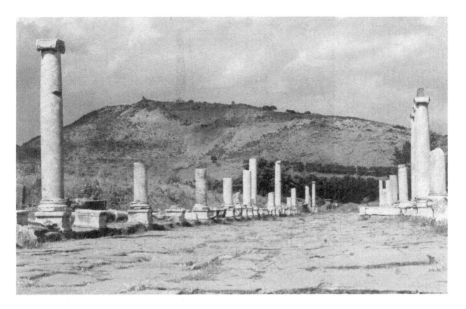

Figure 3.1 The Via Tecta entering the Pergamon Asclepian. One can imagine the booths of energetic merchants lined up on the sides, hawking their votive body parts. (Author's photo, 2005.)

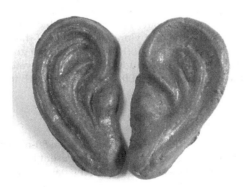

Figure 3.2 Clay-baked votive ears, Circa 200 BC to 200 AD. If the supplicant had an ear problem, these were bought as an offering. Richer patients could buy gold votives. (From Wellcome Library, London, under CC X 4.0.)

gymnasia; theater; an abaton (dream room); and spaces for rituals, festivals, and displays of votives and testimonials.

In the center of the sanctuary itself, there was an area for a large mud bath. Patients stepped down into the bowl-like area and spent time in the paste-like soil. There were two sacred springs next to this area. The muddy supplicant bathed in water and then dressed in a white robe.

15

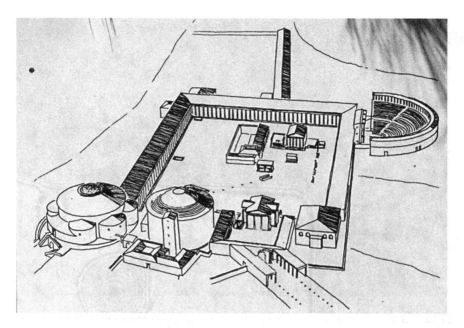

Figure 3.3 Recreated model for the Asclepian Temple at Pergamum (not to scale). The dimensions of the temple complex were enormous. It occupied the equivalent of three American football fields or two World Cup football areas. The lower left round complex was the abaton or dream chamber. The temple is next on the right. It contained a large statue of Asclepius. Next on the right was the propylon or monumental gate. The street, Via Tecta, coming from the city of Pergamum, connected the propylon. To the right of the entrance was a library for which little is known. The dotted line inside the grounds represents the underground cryptoportico. The mud baths and clear water springs were near the middle of the complex. The 3,000-seat theater is atth top right. (From Dosseman, CC BY-SA 4.0, via Wikimedia Commons.)

CRYPTOPORTICO

Adjacent to one of the springs, 12 steps descend into an 80-meter-long underground passage known as the cryptoportico. The present tense is used here since the visitor can still see the stairs and walk the passageway (Figure 3.4). The massive masonry vaults of the cryptoportico are built below ground level, and inside them, it is quiet, dimly lit, and refreshingly cool. Water from the sacred spring would have gently flowed down the steps of the cryptoportico to one side. The sound of these modest falls undoubtedly enhanced the mystic atmosphere. The cryptoportico connected the bathing area to the abaton or dream room. However, as patients walked through the cryptoportico, priests or physicians used the openings in the roof of the tunnel to voice suggestions at the beginning of their dream treatment.

Before their ritual, it is possible that supplicants were given a potion to help them sleep and promote dreams. The abaton was kept in semi-darkness, and flickering lights from perfumed candles accentuated the cult statue of Asclepius. The priests and priestesses, with their hair bound in white fillets, dressed like

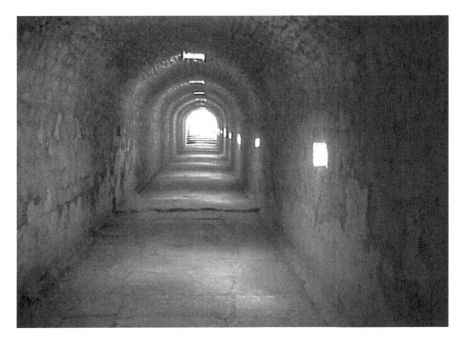

Figure 3.4 The cryptoportico. This stone-lined tunnel led from the mud baths to the abaton. Note the light coming from squares in the ceiling. Priests would have spoken suggestions through the holes. The square patches of light on the wall are sunshine from the ceiling openings. Photo taken in midday. (Author's photo, June 2005.)

Asclepius, circulated among the sleepers and touched them. Supplicants must have dreamed that Asclepius had visited and treated them. While response rates are not recorded for dream therapy, the nature of temple medicine would tend to select only for patients with chronic non-fatal illnesses.

In any case, the purchased votive pieces from the temple entry were laid on the altar of Asclepius upon leaving the sanctuary by grateful worshippers. These gold and clay items were then recycled back to the sellers, and the income used to support the priests and physicians. Criticism of the temple fee system was not lacking. Libanius (314–393 AD) defended the selling of votives, even if the god did not need wealth. He argued the gods were prone to beneficence of their own free will, but that they were even better disposed when petitioned and a fee paid at the temple.[4,5]

Getting to the temple was a significant barrier. Assault by bandits and fear of robbery kept many away. The slow means of ancient travel to the temple prevented attempts by most patients with acute infection or terminal illness. Even if patients with an advanced illness arrived at the temple, they were excluded. Furthermore, the refusal to admit pregnant women about to deliver certainly eliminated the all-too-common problems of fetal and maternal mortality. The selected population allowed inside were those with chronic illnesses. Ultimately, the temple system delivered a powerful placebo (see Chapter 13).

CONCLUSION

The popularity and worship of Asclepius continued into the third century, but then weakened with the rise of Christianity. The Roman emperor Constantine made Christianity a legal religion in 313 AD. The Roman gods lost support. Added to a general climate of decline in paganism, a devastating earthquake destroyed the Asclepian sanctuary at Pergamum in 252 AD.[6]

Galen was ambivalent about Asclepius. In a plea to the deity to heed Emperor Marcus Aurelius, he describes Asclepius as a "demi-god" using the Greek word for "demon" rather than "theos," the word for "god."[7]

Hippocrates and Galen have been pointed to as examples of the development of rational and empirical medicine. In many ways, they were. But side by side, the Asclepian system of treatment flourished. At its best, temple medicine dispensed placebos; at its worst, it continued a system of magic.

NOTES

1 Hart G. *Asclepius: The God of Medicine*. London: Royal Society of Medicine Press; 2000, p. 83.

2 Ibid, p. 179.

3 Freely JP. *Architectural Guides for Travelers: Classical Turkey*. New York: Penguin Books; 1990, pp. 27–41.

4 Avalos H. *Health Care and the Rise of Christianity*. Peabody, MA: Hendrickson Publishers; 1999, p. 92. DOI: 10.1177/004057360205800414

5 The numerous gods to be propitiated in polytheism is quite cumbersome. See Avalos, pp. 20–22. The practice of polytheism still exists.

6 Christianity differed from pagan worship of the Roman gods. The capricious Roman gods existed only to be cajoled into helping the human population with winning battles, rain for crops, or healing. There was little or no ethical obligation required of the supplicant.

7 Hart, p. 5.

4 Authority as Proof

What can we take away from Egyptian medicine? The early deterioration of the intestines after death impressed the ancient Nile dwellers. This led to speculation about the WHDW, or the rotten stuff, spreading throughout the body to cause disease.

The Egyptian response to corruption was cleanliness, even to the extent of shaved heads. Certainly, hygiene has its virtue and helps minimize skin diseases and lice infestations. The ideology went too far in supposing that frequent enemas help get rid of the rotten stuff.

Egyptian medicine was suffused with magical incantations. Every culture has its amulets and talismans. Amulets ward off disease-producing demons, while talismans carry beneficial forces. Archaeologists have discovered thousands of Horus eye amulets in Egypt and hundreds of molds from which the amulets were made.

It is of interest that the most common ingredient in Egyptian wound salves, honey, is an inhibitor of the bacterium, *Staphylococcus aureus*. This suggests different wound ointments were compared to determine which helped wounds heal best. Still, no empirical work is reported.

One is hard put to recognize "science" in Ancient Egyptian medicine, at least by today's standards. It is unclear whether there was any basis for comparing one treatment to another or in ascertaining the best approach. The Nile dwellers were pragmatic, and their fear of the gods prevented them from prying into matters not practical.

Greece gradually took over Egypt in the period 700–300 BC and developed a renowned academic center in Alexandria. The Egyptians were clearly responsible for transmitting their ideas about the rotten stuff to the Greeks. The Ancient Greeks readily attributed their developing viewpoint to the Egyptians.

The humoral theory of Greek physicians reigned central to medical thought for 2,000 years. It was a refined and expanded version of the metu and WHDW. The humoral theory, developed by Galen, presents a logical framework for understanding and treating disease. The Galenic physician withdrew blood to balance the humors and remedy inflammation. The underlying ideas, however, were fundamentally flawed.[1]

The humoral theory reappears when a modern doctor treats the chemistry of the blood as an end in itself. Euboxic ("u box ik") is modern medical slang that refers to all the blood tests of a patient returning in the "normal" range. Physicians, especially younger ones, get frustrated when euboxic patients have the temerity to die.

The chapter on the Asclepian art was included to show that medicine in the ancient world was not all "rational." With more than 500 temples across the Roman Empire, a certain amount of medical care was accomplished. But given the exclusion of acutely ill people and pregnant women, only a fraction of the afflicted were taken care of. There are no follow-up data yet discovered to help us know the effectiveness of Asclepian medicine.

BLOODLETTING

Was there proof that bloodletting helped patients? The Galenic physician withdrew blood to treat and fight inflammation. Galen's understanding of inflammation was the same as ours. In the first century AD, the Roman encyclopedist, Celsus, delineated four signs of inflammation: calor, dolor, rubor, and tumor: or heat, pain, redness, and swelling.[2]

DOI: 10.1201/9781003324058-4

Venesection clearly gave symptomatic relief. Physicians that took blood were not inobservant. The short-term effects appear anti-inflammatory. The swelling would abate with a reduction in pain, redness, and heat. Modern authors tend to place the positive effects as placebo (see Chapter 13) or even allege universal harm from venesection. But where is the evidence of harm? There are precious few data.[3]

The Galenic physician often defined disease as a general construct, such as inflammation or fever. These findings are classified as signs of a particular disease by a modern physician. A disease now has many diagnostic elements to distinguish it from another.

The humoral theory may sound tedious to the modern reader. In reality, it was a simple construct. Grasping Hippocratic theory is needed to make sense of historical writings since it is the basis for understanding disease in historical writings until the early twentieth century.

Examination of a famous case will be helpful here. The final illness of George Washington involved bloodletting.

THE DEATH OF GEORGE WASHINGTON

On December 12, 1799, George Washington, only 30 months after retiring as president, spent most of the day on horseback. In frigid rain and snow, he was supervising activities on his Mount Vernon estate. Late for dinner, Washington remained in his damp clothes throughout the meal. During the day, he had "taken a cold" and was mildly hoarse.[4]

At two the next morning, he awoke with mild rasping. At 6 a.m., a fever started. His throat pain and respiratory distress worsened. He could barely swallow, and speaking was difficult.

His aide, Colonel Tobias Lear, sent for an Edinburgh-trained physician, James Craik, and the estate's overseer and trained bloodletter, George Rawlins. Washington instructed Rawlins to begin bloodletting at 7:30 a.m. Fourteen ounces were removed, and the president asked Rawlins to take more. Lear gave Washington a mixture of molasses, vinegar, and butter, which nearly brought on fatal choking.

Dr. Craik arrived at 9 a.m. As an old friend and physician, he was a frequent visitor to Mt. Vernon. The two men had fought together in the French and Indian Wars. Craik removed 18 ounces of blood at 9:30 a.m. and a similar amount at 11 a.m.

After the third bloodletting, Washington sat up in a chair and began to try to drip vinegar down his throat. Choking again, he stopped. He then rose and paced about the bedroom. This was followed by sitting upright again in a chair for two hours. Returning to bed, the president could not find a comfortable position.

A second physician, Elisha Dick, arrived at 3 p.m. Dr. Dick argued that additional bleeding might weaken Washington too much. Nevertheless, Craik oversaw a fourth bloodletting with the removal of 32 ounces of blood. After this, the president's condition appeared to rally. He was able to swallow. He examined his will.[5]

After 8 p.m., Washington's condition began to deteriorate. Poultices were applied. Around 10 p.m., Washington whispered burial instructions to Lear. At 10:20 a.m., December 14, 1799, George Washington died. The most probable cause was from suffocation.

In retrospect, the diagnosis would now be referred to as "acute bacterial epiglottitis" (i.e., infection of the voice box), but such a term did not exist at the turn of the nineteenth century. The attending physicians recognized the inflammation (i.e., redness and swelling) that caused the narrow throat in their 67-year-old patient. The standard approach, consistent with the humoral theory of the day, was to remove blood by phlebotomy. Washington urged the bedside attendants to start and repeat the bloodletting.

Over the next 12 hours of illness, around 80 ounces (2,400 mL) of blood was removed from George Washington. The only dispute among the physicians was how much blood should be taken. While the physicians never stated their rationale, the reasoning would have been the reduction of inflammation induced by phlebotomy. They were also treating "fever." These were general signs of illness that warranted a Galenic therapeutic attack. It would be another 70–100 years before specific diseases would become the treatment target of the aiming physician.

Did the withdrawal of 2,400 mL of blood cause the president's death? Some historians have thought so. A 6 foot 3 inch (191 cm), 220-pound (100 kg) man has about 6,300 mL of blood in his body. It seems doubtful that losing 2,400 mL would have been a direct or indirect cause of death, given the excellent functional capacity of George Washington.[6]

While historical sources note Washington was treated with the standard therapeutic approach for his time, the regimen is identical to one laid down by Galen 1,500 years earlier,

> If there is no urgency, [one should] make the first bloodletting rather small, and perform a second one—and, if you like, a third—later. Thus, in cases where extensive evacuation is called for, but the faculties are not strong, it is appropriate to divide up the evacuation, as you must have seen me doing in patients who have a plethos of somewhat crude humors. After I have let a little blood, I immediately give some melicratum,[7] nicely cooked. ... After this I take blood again, sometimes on the same day, sometimes on the next; at which time I again give one of the drugs mentioned, in the same way, and remove blood once more; and on the third day I repeat the same process twice. When, however, there is a plethos of seething blood, enkindling a severe fever, there is need for copious evacuation. One must strive to evacuate this blood to the point of fainting, keeping an eye on the strength of the faculties.[8]

EVALUATION OF BLOODLETTING

The proof for or against bloodletting was sparse. In 1836, Pierre Louis published a monograph entitled, *Researches on the Effects of Bloodletting in Some Inflammatory Diseases*. Louis was a meticulous clinician in Paris with ample case records. The 77 patients selected for his bloodletting analysis were a homogeneous group with a well-characterized form of pneumonia. They had all been in good health at the time of the first symptoms of their disease.[9]

After establishing the timing of the onset of the symptoms in each patient, Louis analyzed the duration of the disease and the frequency of death by the timing of the first bloodletting. He grouped patients by early bleeding (days 1–4 of the illness) or late venesection (days 5–9). This resulted in two groups of 41 and 36 patients, which were of comparable average age (41 and 38 years, respectively).

What did Louis find when he compared the evolution of the disease among the two groups? He determined that the duration of disease was an average of three days shorter in those who had been bled early compared with those who had been bled late. However, "three sevenths" (44 %) of the patients who had been bled early died compared to "only one fourth" (25 %) of those bled late, a result Louis remarked was "startling and apparently absurd."[10]

Despite his results, Louis asserted the therapy was beneficial for severe cases of pneumonia,

> I will add that bloodletting, notwithstanding its influence, is limited, should not be neglected in inflammations which are severe…both on account of its influence on the state of the diseased organ; and because in shortening the duration of the disease, it diminishes the chance of secondary lesions.[11]

What we want to know is what would have happened to a control group not receiving venesection. Moreover, Louis failed to use the solid criterion of mortality, rather than the softer endpoint of recovery. His attitude was, "Don't confuse me with the facts, I want to conclude that venesection is helpful."

Despite the discordance between his results and conclusion, Louis's recommendations stood for more than a century in the treatment of severe pneumonia. The iconic medical textbook by William Osler in its 14th edition in 1942 still had not changed the advice about bleeding in pneumonia.[12,13]

BETTER OR WORSE THAN DOING NOTHING?

In any case, none of the ancient systems had any means to compare the efficacy of a given therapy. For the modern reader, how do we know that any ancient treatment was better than doing nothing? Or that the treatment given was superior to any other? Obvious questions not addressed in Egyptian, Greek, or Asclepian medicine.

There is an innate desire when someone is sick to "do something." Consequently, there are "treatments" for every disease. The key question is, "Do any of the treatments improve the patient?"

Simply put, a better outcome can be recognized when it is compared to not giving any therapy to a similar person with the same disease. Without comparison, how do we know whether the patient is better or worse?

Proof. We seek proof of efficacy. Efficacy is the maximum beneficial effect that can be achieved with an intervention. The sources of proof for two millennia were either authoritarian or personal. First, the authority of Galen. His ideas reigned for 1,700 years from the third century to the twentieth century. One merely cited Galen as proof that a therapy was best.

The second major source of authority came from the pagan gods. What greater proof could there be than to have a god tell you? Galen complained, "[E]ven among ourselves in Pergamum, we see that those being treated by the god obey him when he orders them, as he does on many occasions, not to drink [alcohol] for 15 days, while they obey none of the physicians who give this prescription."[14]

Then there is the judgment of the patient and physician. Certainly, patients can and should attempt to evaluate their therapy. But subjective feelings of processes inside their body may not be accurate. And if experience is fallacious for a physician's self-treatment, it is even more so for a patient encountering a disease for the first time.[15]

Medical students gain knowledge from their teachers. They have been taught anatomy and physiology as a basis for judging signs and symptoms. But, if the anatomy and physiology they have learned are imperfect, then their conclusions are defective.

The reader grasps what illness is from the patient's viewpoint—an undesirable set of symptoms that are subjective. On the other hand, disease is the objective side of the problem. Disease manifests itself as a disorder in function or form of cells or organs. Disease presents tangible signs for an observer, such as a fever or jaundice (yellow skin).

There are two confounders in judging outcome. One, the natural history of disease. That is, what happens if we do nothing? "If you take two of these pills a day for your cold, you will be cured in seven days. If you do not take the pills, you will be well in a week."

Second, there is the placebo effect. A placebo effect is a substance or treatment (such as a sugar pill) known to have no influence on a disease. Yet, when a placebo is given to patients with acute or chronic illness, about a third of sufferers with almost any disease show an abatement of symptoms for days to weeks before evidence of their disease relapses or abates spontaneously. The placebo effect of temple medicine must have been substantial.

These sources of authority or physician and personal judgment are still with us today. They are not necessarily detrimental. But the greatest progress in medical treatment has been made with numerical comparison. But before the simplicity and elegance of numbers, a few chapters are needed to bridge the Galenic world and the twenty-first century. Then, how modern quacks have duped the unwitting.

NOTES

1 The author's grandfather, Frederick Albert Hand, related how as a boy, around the year 1919, he was reluctant to go to a small-town doctor in Nebraska. All this doctor gave for any internal illness was a laxative!

2 Every first-year medical student is taught these descriptors.

3 There are a few diseases where periodic bloodletting is beneficial such as hemochromatosis—a genetic disease where the intestines absorb too much iron, and this leads to diabetes, heart and liver failure.

4 Knox JHM. The medical history of George Washington, his physicians, friends, and advisors. *Bulletin of the Institute of the History of Medicine* 1933;1; pp. 174–91.

5 Morens DM. Death of a president. *New England Journal of Medicine* 1999;341; pp. 1845–9. DOI: 10.1056/NEJM199912093412413

6 The author is a gastroenterologist who has treated more than a thousand patients with gastrointestinal bleeding. Mortality during gastrointestinal bleeding is very much related to the patient's functional (i.e., cardiopulmonary health). Given that he had been riding a horse all day, we can infer he had a good functional capacity. On the other hand, reports agree he could swallow almost nothing and his respiratory distress was great. These latter findings suggest suffocation was the principal cause.

7 Melicratum was a fermented or unfermented beverage of honey and water. Galen would add hyssop or other herbs to the drink.

8 Brain P. *Galen on Bloodletting: A Study of the Origins, Development and Validity of his Opinions, with a Translation of the Three Works*. London: Cambridge University Press; 1986, pp. 85–8.

9 Morabia A. Pierre-Charles-Alexandre Louis and the evaluation of bloodletting. *Journal of Royal Society of Medicine* 2006;99; pp. 158–60. DOI: 10.1258/jrsm.99.3.158

10   Louis PCA. *Researches on the Effects of Bloodletting in Some Inflammatory Diseases: And on the Influence of Tartarized Antimony and Vesication in Pneumonitis.* Hilliard: Gray; 1836, p. 9.

11   Louis, p. 23.

12   Thomas D. The demise of bloodletting. *Journal of the Royal College of Physicians of Edenborough* 2014;44; pp. 72–7. DOI: 10.4997/JRCPE.2014.117

13   Penicillin, available in the mid-1940s, was so effective for pneumonia that it supplanted any other therapy.

14   Hart G. *Asclepius: The God of Medicine.* London: Royal Society of Medicine Press; 2000, p. 83.

15   Though the old cliché is still true, "The doctor who treats himself has a fool for a patient."

5 Andreas Vesalius and Keen Observation

The work of Andreas Vesalius of Brussels (Figure 5.1) represents one of the greatest treasures of Western civilization. His masterpiece, the *De Humani Corporis Fabrica*, hereafter referred to as the *Fabrica*, published in Basel, Switzerland, in 1543, established with startling suddenness a revolution in observational research.

Born in Brussels in 1514 and dying in 1564, the year of Michelangelo's death and Shakespeare's birth, the life of Vesalius occurs during the Renaissance. Among his contemporaries were Leonardo Da Vinci, Raphael, and Cervantes.

Vesalius was the first physician to obtain his own observation of the human body and to turn those observations into bold questioning of Galenic authority. The Greco-Roman foundation began to crack under Vesalius's appeal to visual proof.

The likely lifelong goal of Vesalius was to become a court physician to the Spanish emperor, Charles V. This thesis appeals, as it unifies his biography and provides a rational account for his abrupt movements.

For as far back as his great-grandfather, John, the family of Vesalius served as medical advisors for the Hapsburg dynasty. John served as physician to the Duke of Burgundy. The court physicians of the day focused on the influence of astrology on medical conditions. His father, also named Andreas, served as apothecary to the emperor, Charles V. His father's library was extensive, and Vesalius became an avid reader and inhabitant of the family library.

In 1528, Vesalius entered the University of Louvain, where he continued reading medieval writers on science. His interest in anatomy was already evident as he began dissecting small animals.

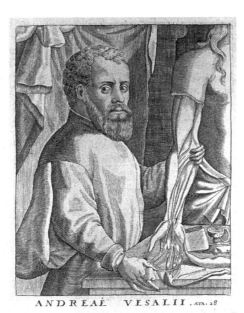

ANDREAE VESALII . ÆTA. 28

Figure 5.1 Woodcut picture of Andreas Vesalius. This is the only known portrait of the famous anatomist. (From Wellcome Library, London. Attribution International 4.0 [CC x 4.0].)

DOI: 10.1201/9781003324058-5

In 1533, Vesalius, now ready for formal medical education, set out for the University of Paris. The medical school required knowledge of anatomy but did not have human dissections or practical teachers of anatomy. Candidates gained their knowledge from textbooks, where the ancient teachings of Galen remained supreme.

The *Cemetery of the Innocents* provided bone specimens. Reconstruction of the city wall of Paris in 1186 had disinterred many fragmented skeletons into charnel houses.

There Vesalius and his fellow students found,

> An abundant supply when I first studied the bones...and having learned by long and tiring observation, we, even blindfolded, dared at times to wager with our companions, and in half-an-hour no bone could be offered us... which we could not identify by touch. This had to be done the more zealously by us who desired to learn inasmuch as there was a great lack of the assistance of teachers in this part of medicine.[1]

UNIVERSITY OF PADUA

Vesalius left Paris when war broke out between France and Spain. He eventually landed in Italy, where he entered the University of Padua. A description of Padua is necessary, since Vesalius, and the subject of our second biography, William Harvey, trained there. The city of Padua today is still rich with features that would have greeted the observant eye of Vesalius. It is 30 miles west of Venice and stands in the plain at the foot of the Euganean hills. Near the center of the city, close to the Palace of Justice, is the old university, the focus of Vesalius's studies.

As a university, Padua was the offspring of Bologna, where in 1170 AD, the first guilds of students were formed. Contrary to the modern era, students in the High Middle Ages were the source of academic power. The students decided the content of the curriculum and invited the professors to teach. In 1222 AD, disputes in Bologna between students, faculty, and local authorities caused such tensions that waves of students left for other cities, including 3,000 who left for Padua.

In 1537, Vesalius was granted permission to perform a human dissection before his eager fellow students, the first demonstration of human anatomy the city had witnessed in 18 years. Human dissection had become well accepted in Europe by the sixteenth century, particularly in Italy. The availability of bodies was limited, as only executed criminals were used, necessitating the rare demonstration of dissection to a large group.

Contrary to myth (i.e., false claim), the medieval church did not prohibit human dissection.[2]

> Although the church did not prohibit human dissection in the early Middle Ages, there is no evidence of its practice. In the late thirteenth century, we find the first evidence of the opening of human bodies by medical men, in connection with municipally mandated autopsies, to determine the cause of death in the interests of criminal justice or public health.[3,4]

The use of human bodies for anatomical training does not appear to have taken place anywhere in the world until around the year 1300 in the Italian city of Bologna. In the last two millennia, apart from the recording of a few human dissections in Islamic countries during the Middle Ages (Circa 800–1200 AD), there has been no evidence of autopsies re-starting again in the Middle East until recently. China and Japan avoided the practice completely well into the twentieth century. Only in Western civilization was human anatomical dissection performed after 1300 AD.

The reader can review the title page of Vesalius's *Fabrica*, published in 1543, and determine for themselves that there are numerous clergymen in attendance for the anatomical dissection. Their presence indicates approval.

On December 5, 1537, the faculty of the University of Padua, after examining Vesalius, granted him the degree of doctor of medicine cum ultima diminution (with the highest distinction). On the following day, after performing a dissection, he was nominated as professor of surgery, which at that time bore the responsibility of teaching anatomy as well. Why or how Vesalius obtained such early recognition, despite his youthful age of 23 years, is unknown, but he must have made a profound impression on his professors.

With characteristic energy, the young professor began his academic duties with success. The standard procedure at the time was for the professor to sit aloof in a chair on an elevated platform and read the description of the dissection that was carried out by one of his underlings. Not so for Vesalius. He stepped off the throne and performed it himself amid his lecture at the table side.

How aggressive was Vesalius in pursuing his opportunities for dissection? A note written by him at age 32, looking back at his younger days, says in part,

> I shall no longer bother to petition the judges to delay the day of an execution of a criminal to a time suitable for my dissection of his body, nor shall I advise the medical students to observe where someone has been buried or urge them to note the diseases of their teachers' patients so that they might later seize their bodies. I shall not keep in my bedroom for several weeks bodies taken from graves or given me after public execution, nor shall I put up with the bad temper of sculptors and painters who made me more miserable than did the bodies I was dissecting. However, too young to gain financially from the art and wishing to learn and to advance our common studies, I readily and cheerfully supported all these things.[5,6]

Vesalius's observations often disagreed with incontrovertible ancient authority, and this audacity drew crowds of learned men eager to dispute with him. Instead, many went away convinced by the visible evidence demonstrated by Vesalius. Others, though, when shown visible proof, replied with the quaint response that if current anatomy differed from Galen, it must be that men had degenerated their anatomy since ancient time!

To clarify his demonstrations, Vesalius introduced huge charts detailing human anatomy. Oddly enough, illustration of human anatomy was unheard of. Opposition arose not only over content but even the visual method. His students however quickly grasped the superiority of the visual aids for learning. His six large charts were quickly plagiarized throughout Europe, forcing Vesalius to publish them. The six charts were published without title in 1538 but are now known as the *Tabulae Anatomicae Sex*.

In 1540, Vesalius was invited to Bologna by the university faculty to demonstrate dissection and lecture. The significance of this event is that it produced the only surviving firsthand notes of a student, Baldasar Heseler, who took detailed minutes of the lecture and the response of the class. Heseler was a German student with a bachelor's degree in theology received while studying under Martin

Luther at the University of Wittenberg. The study of theology was a common pre-medical subject for sixteenth-century physicians.

The other prosector during the lectures was the local professor and convinced Galenist, Matteus Curtius. Heseler made no secret that he disapproved of Curtius's "vain glorious demeanor." The dissection involved three bodies and took place in the Church of San Francesco in Bologna.[7]

One duty of any sixteenth-century surgical teacher was to teach the technique of venesection for bloodletting. Curtius agreed with Galen, who had taught that in pleurisy, bloodletting was to be done on the affected side of the body in pleurisy, while Vesalius agreed that either was acceptable. Furthermore, the young visiting professor appealed to the evidence derived from dissection for support of his therapeutic recommendation. Heseler records the following volatile exchange between the two professors, where we pick up Vesalius saying,

> "'Now,' he said, excellentissime Domine, here we have our bodies. We shall judge whether I have made an error. Now we want to look at this and leave Galen, for I acknowledge that I have said, if it is permissible to say so, that here Galen is in the wrong, because he did not know the position of the vein without pair in the human body, which is the same today just as it was in his time.
>
> Curtius answered smiling, for Vesalius, choleric as he was, was animated, 'No,' he said, 'Domine, we must not leave Galen, because he always well understood everything, and consequently, we also follow him. Do you know how to interpret Hippocrates better than Galen?'
>
> Vesalius answered, 'I do not say so, but I show you here in these two bodies the vein without the pair, how it nourishes all the lower ribs, except the two upper ones, in which there is no pleurisy. For always here,' he knocked with his hands against the middle of the chest, 'occurs inflammation and pleurisy, not at the two upper ribs. Consequently, as this vein is also distant from the heart, as you observe by three fingers' breadth, it will always be in pleurisy, and all morbus lateralis [it would] be better to bleed from this vein only; or it ought to be no difference from what part bleeding is done, because the ribs are nourished exclusively by this vein."

Curtius replied:	'I am no anatomista, but there can also be other veins nourishing the ribs and the muscles besides these.'
	'Where, please,' Vesalius said, 'show them to me.'
	Curtius said, 'Do you want to deny the ducts of Nature?'
	'Oh,' Vesalius said, 'you want to talk about things not visible and concealed. I again talk about what is visible.'
Curtius answered:	'Indeed, I always deal with what is most obvious. Domine, you do not well understand Hippocrates and Galen on this.'
Vesalius replied:	'It is quite true, because I am not so old a man as you are.'
Curtius said:	'Not at all, Domine.' And thus, Curtius left."[8]

Heseler then comments that with much quarreling and scoffing, they attacked each other. At the end of the demonstration, he records Curtius asked Vesalius not to be angry with him.[4]

BASEL AND FABRICA

Over the next five years, the young professor compiled his monumental seven-volume work on anatomy. He engaged artists to perfect his drawings and wrote extensively about the content of hundreds of plates depicting human anatomy.

In 1543, he took his precious proofs over the Alps to Basel, Switzerland, the center of European printing, and oversaw production of the delicate illustrations. Little is known of Vesalius's life in Basel. Presumably, he was occupied with proofreading.

During his stay, however, several chroniclers recorded a dramatic crime. It was an incident related to Vesalius, in that he was to dissect the body of the executed criminal and construct a skeleton from its bones.[9] Briefly, the first and still married wife of a habitual criminal discovered her husband had a second wife and confronted him about it. The next day, the bigamist waited to ambush his first wife in a field. When she stopped to rest, he attacked her with sword and knife and inflicted many wounds, nearly cutting off her left arm. A manhunt ensued, and the faithless husband was soon apprehended. He was tried and convicted.

With the publication of the book, the breadth and detail of Vesalius's *Fabrica* stunned the scientific world. In it, Vesalius pointed out the errors Galen had made because the latter had dissected dogs or other animals rather than humans. Galen believed the liver gave rise to the blood, the uterus had multiple channels, and the pituitary poured its secretions into the nose. Based upon the anatomy of sheep, the blood supply at the base of the brain for centuries was presumed to be a mass of blood vessels, not the single collateral blood vessel of humans. The modern reader perusing his plates is impressed with the accuracy and vitality of his drawings of the human body (Figure 5.2).

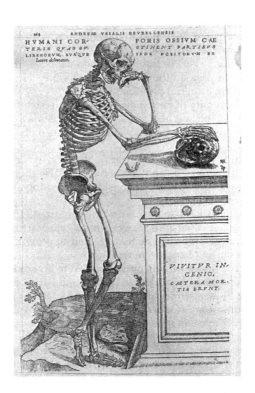

Figure 5.2 A skeleton soliloquizing to a skull. The Latin motto on the tomb, *"Vivitur ingenio, cactera mortis erunt"*—"Genius lives on, all else is mortal."

That Vesalius dared to correct the ancient master was too much for some. Jacob Sylvanius, Vesalius's former anatomy teacher at the University of Paris, wrote in an open letter to the emperor,

> I implore his Imperial Majesty to punish severely, as he deserves, this monster born and bred in his own house, this worst example of ignorance, ingratitude, arrogance and impiety, to suppress him so that he may not poison the rest of Europe with his pestilential breath.[10]

Though Vesalius is often portrayed as quick-tempered, his later description of his lost reply to his former teacher reveals a steadiness as he responded to his critics,

> These men could not believe that the father of medicine had made such mistakes in the anatomical books he felt he had written with so much care and accuracy, the more so since it was a subject in which he had acquired greater authority than anyone else, even during his own lifetime. Gradually, however, they began to change their attitude, and there was not one among them who, with the cadaver before him, could continue to defend Galen. However reluctantly, they came to put more faith in their eyes than in the words of Galen. It is my hope that eventually Sylvius, too, will change his mind as he reads what I have written, and that he will not deny me his good will and friendship.[11]

THE IMPERIAL COURT

After the printing was done, Vesalius hastened to the Imperial Court of Charles V to present his masterpiece dedicated to the emperor. With its generous size of 11 by 16 inches, an imperial purple silk velvet binding, and 700 pages displaying the finest illustrations ever contained in a medical book, the special copy of the *Fabrica* must have impressed the emperor enormously. He soon appointed Vesalius as an attending imperial physician.[12]

Vesalius left the University of Padua and ceased his research and teaching. His abrupt departure at the height of his academic career is a puzzle. The most facile explanation for his career change was that he was merely achieving a lifelong ambition.

Vesalius penned in 1546, three years after publication of the *Fabrica*, that the many unfounded criticisms of it "gnawed at his soul." He therefore escaped to the Imperial Court, where "I would not consider publishing anything new even if I wanted to."

Nevertheless, Vesalius's fame led to consultation requests from the aristocratic class of Europe. His attendance at the famous head injury (from a jousting event) of Henry II or the strange illness of the teenage heir-apparent, Don Carlos, of Spain, has been the subject of extensive writing.

After 20 years at court, Vesalius abruptly decided to accept the now illustrious and vacant chair of anatomy at Padua. He returned to Padua full of enthusiasm, but before resuming his academic duties, Vesalius decided to undergo a pilgrimage to Palestine for unknown reasons.

Incredulous writers have advanced numerous theories about why Vesalius left for a pilgrimage. One plausible reason is that Vesalius fell ill in the King's Court, and his life was despaired of. He made a vow to go to the Holy Land in case of his recovery. Upon recuperation, he did so. Shipwrecked upon his return, Vesalius died on October 15, 1564, at age 49. He was buried on the Mediterranean island of Zante.

What further anatomical advances Vesalius could have made upon his sequel to Padua can only be guessed. He might have pre-empted the discovery of the circulation of the blood, finally advanced by William Harvey in 1628. Vesalius might have accelerated medical thinking by a century.

Centuries later, William Osler, the father of American medicine, described *Fabrica* as the "greatest book in medicine."[13] Beyond the contribution of his beautiful book, his courage to identify and correct mistakes considered correct for more than a thousand years is his legacy to modern medical science. The dogmatic aspect of classical medicine was finally breached.

NOTES

1 Vesalius A, Saunders JM, O'Malley CD. *The Illustrations from the Works of Andreas Vesalius of Brussels: With Annotations and Translations, a Discussion of the Plates and their Background, Authorship and Influence, and a Biographical Sketch of Vesalius.* Cleveland, OH: Courier Corporation; 1950, p. 14.

2 The reader is referred to Katherine Park's essay in *Galileo Goes to Jail and other Myths about Science and Religion.*[3]

3 Park K. Myth [number] 5. That the Medieval Church Prohibited Human Dissection. In: Numbers R, ed. *Galileo Goes to Jail and Other Myths about Science and Religion.* Cambridge, MA: Harvard University Press; 2009: location 14%–15%.

4 The Ancient Greeks and Romans avoided human dissection. Their aversion seems rooted in the belief that corpses were ritually unclean. Early Christianity broke from this idea of pollution and embraced tombs as holy places and the bodies of the dead as objects of veneration. The author has wandered through the Christian catacombs outside Rome. The celebration of the underground cemetery is shown by the many works of art in the catacombs, which date as early as the third century AD.

5 Friedman M. *Medicine's 10 Greatest Discoveries.* New Haven, CT: Yale University Press; 1998, p. 4.

6 Bodies in his bedroom for several weeks? Smell? How could one sleep?

7 The venue should dispel any final doubt about the ecclesiastical attitude toward human dissection.

8 Eriksson R. Andreas *Vesalius' First Public Anatomy at Bologna, 1540. An Eyewitness Report by Baldasar Heseler Medicinæ Scolaris, Together with his Notes on Matthaeus Curtius' Lectures on Anatomia Mundini.* Stockholm: Almqvist & Wiksells; 1959, p. 273.

9 His remains have the distinction of being the oldest existing anatomical specimen in the world. The skeleton can still be seen in the Museum of the Anatomical Institute of the University of Basel.

10 De Humani Corporis Fabrica: Andreas Vesalius. https://www.codex99.com/anatomy/45.html (accessed August 1, 2018).

11 O'Malley CD. *Andreas Vesalius of Brussels, 1514–1564.* Berkeley, CA: University of California Press; 1964, p. 219–20.

12 Unfortunately, the last original copy of this special imperial edition perished in Belgium during World War I.

13 Friedman, p. 3.

6 William Harvey Counts Heartbeats

William Harvey's publication in 1628, *Motion of the Heart*, illuminated for the first time the circulation of the blood. This movement was a topic of ignorance for thousands of years. His keen observations and simple logic established a new way of thinking in biology.

Harvey was born on April 1, 1578, to middle-class English farm parents, Thomas and Joan Harvey. His parents rose to lower gentry through economic success. As a result, William Harvey found himself, at age 15, entering Caius (pronounced "Keys") College in Cambridge. John Caius founded the college in 1567 and was a classmate of Andreas Vesalius at the University of Padua. Caius and the famous anatomist shared living quarters and dissections together.

Upon his return to England, Caius promoted the study of human anatomy through dissection. While Caius was not the earliest professor to perform human dissection in England, he was the first to institute them regularly. He obtained a Charter of Anatomies from Queen Elizabeth in 1565, whereby each fellow of the Royal College of Physicians gave lectures on anatomy. Each took a turn and was liable to pay fines if he did not do so. While an undergraduate, Harvey would not have studied medicine directly. However, Caius College was the best place for a serious young man interested in science or medicine. Short in stature, Harvey's eyes were full of spirit and his hair raven black.

After graduation, Harvey enrolled at the University of Padua in January 1600. In August 1600, he was elected councilor of the English Nation. This election contrasts the different organizations in early Italian universities. Padua was a studia or student university where undergraduates controlled the employment of their teachers. Students were enrolled according to their countries in groups called nations. Each nation elected its own representative. Harvey's election so soon after his arrival in 1600, and his re-election the following two years, reflects the prompt and persistent esteem of his countrymen.[1]

Harvey graduated as a doctor of medicine from the University of Padua in 1602. When he returned to England, Harvey carried with him the open inquiry atmosphere of the University of Padua.

In 1604, Harvey married Elizabeth Browne, whose father was a physician to Queen Elizabeth and King James I. Of Harvey's wife, we know little. They were childless. She did possess a parrot as a longtime pet, which she allowed to perch on her shoulder. According to Harvey, it was a "handsome bird and famous talker." The death of the parrot caused both Harveys "great sorrow." William performed a postmortem and discovered a nearly complete egg in its oviduct.

Harvey was appointed as overseeing physician at St. Bartholomew's Hospital in 1609. His pay was £25 per annum. The hospital for the poor was already 486 years old at this point, but the office of physician had only existed for 41 years.[2] As overseer, he saw ambulatory patients of the hospital once a week in the Great Hall. At the appointed time, he sat at a table and wrote his prescriptions with inkpot and quill pen. Beside him stood the matron and the apothecary. Examination of each patient was brief, and more time was taken writing the prescription, as there were generally five to ten ingredients. He then went to the ward to see the bedridden patients. Finally, his duties included overseeing three surgeons. In Harvey's time, both the education and status of surgeons were inferior to physicians.

From 1612 to 1628, Harvey gave the required lectures on anatomy for the Royal College of Physicians. The lectures were given in six-year cycles, centered on one section of the body, followed by a dissection. He must have

DOI: 10.1201/9781003324058-6

enjoyed lecturing since his 12 years went far beyond the number needed for fulfilling his duty. Copies of his lecture notes are available from those years, and some antecedents to his famous publication can be detected. However, since his ideas on the heart were so radical, Harvey himself said that prior to 1628, he had discussed and demonstrated the anatomical truths to only a few private friends.

THE HEART BEFORE HARVEY

The circulation of blood with the heart as pump is taken for granted by the modern reader. But what was the prevailing belief about the function of the heart prior to Harvey? To enlarge the Galenic idea from Chapter 2 on life force (Figure 2.2), it was held that ingested food was "concocted" (digested by heat) in the stomach. The steam rose as a vapor through the mesenteric vessels to the liver, where it was transformed to venous blood. From the liver, the venous blood was transported through the veins to the periphery of the body for nourishment.

At the periphery, the veins became smaller and smaller until their thread-like ends were converted into flesh. The various parts of the body destroyed the blood (red blood cells were not demonstrated until 50 years later with the microscope) as the nutrients were utilized. Venous blood moved from the liver into the right side of the heart, where some of it went into the pulmonary artery to nourish the lungs, and some passed through imagined holes in the intraventricular septum into the left ventricle.

Inspired air was drawn into the lungs, passed through the pulmonary vein into the left ventricle, and was concocted like milk in a saucepan by the left ventricle into arterial blood. Some of the arterial blood went back into the lungs and the remainder into the aorta. The arterial system was thought to move less blood than the venous system. The movement of blood throughout the body, whether by veins or arteries, was believed to be relatively slow, like the ebb and flow of the ocean tide.

In the defense of the Galenic paradigm, it was known to the ancients that at autopsy, the liver and right side of the heart are congested with blood; the left ventricle is partly filled with clotted blood; arteries contain air and not blood. Galen and others had merely constructed a model that attempted to account for the foregoing observations. Vesalius could not find the porosities in the intraventricular septum (and neither could anyone else). To explain the visual absence of porosities, Galen and other anatomists had theorized that their effacement was due to postmortem shrinkage of the heart.

HARVEY'S REASONING AND PROOF

Harvey was indebted for part of his new paradigm to another Italian, Realdus Columbus, who provided him with one piece of the puzzle by demonstrating the pulmonary transit of blood.

Columbus's book, *De Re Anatomica*, was published posthumously in 1560. It contained the observation that in living animals, incision of the pulmonary vein as far away as possible from the heart revealed only blood and no air. Columbus also correctly understood that the valves of the heart were to prevent regurgitation of blood. Possessed of these facts—namely, lack of intraventricular porosities, blood in the pulmonary vein, and the true notion about valvular function—Columbus realized Galen was wrong and rightly stated the existence of pulmonary circulation.

Perhaps because of his premature death, Columbus's book caused no firestorm of criticism and seemed to have an insignificant impact on his contemporaries. Harvey, however, knew of it since he copied passages from *De Re Anatomica* into his notes for his anatomy lectures for the College of Physicians in 1616.

Harvey revealed the key to his discovery in *Motion of the Heart*:

> Unless the blood should somehow find its way from the arteries into the veins, and so return to the right side of the heart, I began to think whether there might not be a motion, as it were, in a circle.[3]

However, Harvey was anxious for the opinion of his contemporaries and worried his task was too formidable:

> [My idea was] so novel and unheard of that I not only fear injury to myself from the envy of a few, but I tremble lest I have mankind at large for my enemies.[1]

Concerning the formidable task,

> When I first gave my mind to vivisections, as a means of discovering the motions and uses of the heart, and sought to discover these from actual inspection, and not from the writings of others, I found the task so truly arduous, so full of difficulties, that I was almost tempted to think, with Fracastorius, that the motion of the heart was only to be comprehended by God. For I could neither rightly perceive at first when the systole and when the diastole took place, nor when and where dilation and contraction occurred, by reason of the rapidity of the motion, which in many animals is accomplished in the twinkling of an eye.[4]

Harvey's unique solution to the problem of rapid heart motion was the dying reptilian heart, a superb choice for observing the gradual slowing of cardiac motion.[5] It seems strange no one before him exploited this simple means of overcoming the difficulty of interpreting rapid motion.

Harvey deduced the correct interpretation of systole (contraction of the heart and expulsion of blood outside the heart) and diastole (relaxation and infilling of blood into the heart). His conclusions, although correct, were the exact opposite of the ancient paradigm.

Harvey's principle evidence to support circulation was quantitative; namely, the enormous amount of blood that the heart pumped out in even as short of a period as a half hour. He measured the capacity of the postmortem human heart as containing two ounces (60 mL) and postulated the effective output to be 25% or half an ounce (15 mL) with each beat. Multiplying this output times the number of heartbeats in half an hour, Harvey decided that a thousand half ounces (or nearly four gallons or 16 liters) were sent out into the body in this short time period. He concluded this was a "larger quantity in every case than contained in the whole body." He did not know the total amount of blood in the human body, but he was aware of the amount in similar-sized mammals, such as sheep, since this was common knowledge of butchers. In any case, he argued that even this amount, let alone twice the amount needed in one hour (i.e., 32 liters) or 48 times the amount needed in 24 hours (i.e., 1,536 liters), was infinitely more than what could be provided by the individual's ingestion of food and water during the same period. Thus, Harvey was forced to conclude that blood must circulate around the body and not be consumed by the extremities.

Harvey greatly underestimated *cardiac output* (contemporary terminology for the amount of blood expelled by the heart). Cardiac output is now known to be five to seven liters per minute (or 7,200 to 10,080 liters per day)! Nevertheless, the amount calculated by Harvey was sufficient to carry his point.

Harvey's third and final problem to be solved in *Motion of the Heart* was how blood was sent to the extremities and the way it returned to the heart. Given his prior conclusions, it was necessary that the arteries should be the conduit of blood, but how to get this blood to the veins and thence back to the heart?

Harvey's final bit of genius was to properly interpret the meaning of a commonly performed medical procedure—namely, phlebotomy, or the withdrawal of blood from a vein, usually from an arm. To accomplish a phlebotomy, a tourniquet must be placed on the upper arm tight enough to cause the veins to swell, but not so tight as to obliterate the arterial pulse. When this is done, the veins of the arm engorge. Harvey argued this did not prove that veins brought blood into the arm as was supposed, but rather the opposite—that veins returned blood to the heart, and further, the blood must somehow move from the artery to the vein at the periphery.

The weakness of his latter model, as his critics pointed out, is that he could only hypothesize the presence of tiny channels between the arteries and veins. This invisible channel theory appeared to be inconsistent since it came from a man who (correctly) denied the existence of unseen porosities of the heart's intraventricular septum (as Galen taught). The demonstration of capillaries, as these latter invisible channels were to be called, was accomplished by Antony Leeuwenhoek (Chapter 8), later in the seventeenth century. *Motion of the Heart* contained only four figures (Figure 6.1). With these, Harvey added the simple but elegant observation that when a vein is compressed below a valve and the blood stroked away toward the proximal valve (i.e., the shoulder side), no blood will refill the vein. Conversely, when the blood is emptied between two portions of a vein between two valves, and then the finger is lifted from the distal valve (i.e., hand side), it will be noticed the veins fill immediately, with the blood moving toward the heart.

How was *Motion of the Heart* received? In Harvey's own words,

> Some tear the as yet tender infant (of blood circulation) to bits with their wranglings, as undeserving of birth; others by contrast consider that the offspring ought to be nurtured and cherish it and protect it by their writings. …There are those who cry out that I have striven after the empty glory of vivisections, and they disparage and ridicule with childish levity the frogs, snakes, flies and other lower animals which I have brought onto my stage. Nor do they abstain from scurrilous language.[5]

Harvey's key supporter was Dr. John Argent, the president of the Royal College of Physicians. However, other fellows of the college attacked Harvey's theories with ardor. How could animal experiments prove what was happening in the human? The theory clearly contradicted Galen's theory of humors residing in regional areas of the body. With all this blood rapidly recirculating throughout the body, the pooling of humors was impossible. Harvey challenged his opponents to "see for themselves" and not take his word for it.

The official date of acceptance in the home of his medical studies, Italy, may be 1651, occurred when Giovanni Trulli, physician to the Pope, expounded the doctrine in Rome and acknowledged its author.[6]

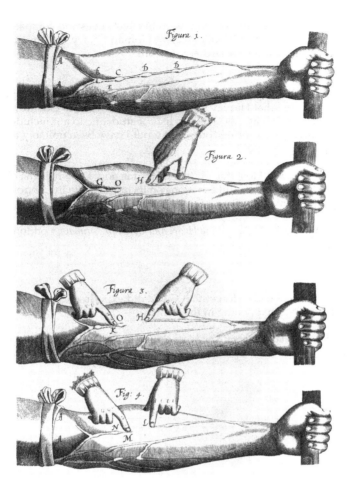

Figure 6.1 Harvey's original figures. He ligatured an arm to distend the veins and their valves and then pressed blood away from the heart and showed the vein remained empty because it was blocked by the valve. (From Wellcome Collection CC by 4.0.)

CONCLUSION

Harvey died in 1657. The great physician is buried in the family chapel at Hempstead.

In calculating cardiac output, Harvey was the first scientist to construct a quantitative argument in describing the function of the body. His paradigm-smashing book provided simple proofs both visual and mathematical to support his model of the circulation of blood. Admirably, he did not use a new technological machine to illuminate muddy waters, as many scientists have done. Rather, he merely looked at everyday knowledge in a new way and reported his observations with clear and simple exposition. A rare thinker.

As we leave Harvey, we can see him with his lively eyes and compact figure standing like a giant with one foot in Galen's Roman library and the other in the operating room of the modern cardiac surgeon.

NOTES

1 The famous Galileo was also at Padua during the Harvey years, and it has been speculated that Harvey knew Galileo. According to Geoffrey Keynes, this seems not the case, as Galileo's lists of students do not include Harvey. Galileo taught engineering courses. It would have been unlikely that Harvey was his student.

2 St. Bartholomew's Hospital, or "Barts" as it is now known, is the oldest hospital in Europe and still functions on its original site in London where it was founded in 1123 AD.

3 Harvey W. *On the Motion of the Heart and Blood in Animals*. London: Bell; 1889, p. 45–6.

4 Harvey, p. 18.

5 These critics seemed to forget that Galen did experiments on animals to assert what was happening in the human.

6 Keele KD. *William Harvey: The Man, the Physician, and the Scientist*. London: Nelson; 1965, p. 165.

7 Smallpox, Edward Jenner, and Numbers

The sudden attack. The fiery torture. The deadly outcome. Smallpox has been the most dreaded disease of all time (Figure 7.1).

To understand what it was like to live before 1800, the would-be historian must be familiar with the danger posed by this life-threatening infection. Everyone in the Old World caught smallpox throughout history, and millions died. It is likely that more human beings have died of smallpox than any other infection in history. Many Egyptian mummies have the tell-tale scarring of the skin.

When infected, as few as one in six victims died. But often nine out of ten. Waves of infection spread through the countryside, creating great anxiety. Infants suffered a high mortality rate. A child was not given a name in frontier America until he or she had survived smallpox, or when they had reached their second birthday.

The earliest record of smallpox in Europe was a plague that began in 165 AD during a Roman military campaign in Mesopotamia. There were so many smallpox casualties, the Imperial army was forced to retreat. Returning soldiers brought the disease to Italy, where it raged for 15 years. At one point, smallpox killed 2,000 victims a day in Rome. As many as ten million people were killed.

Galen (Chapter 2) described the manifestations of this epidemic: "[A] wretched victim suffered from fever, an inflamed throat, vomiting, a black exanthem (pustular) covering an entire body, and…many lesions which changed into ulcers."

In the fifteenth century, the French began calling the new disease of syphilis *la grosse verole* ("great-pox" in English). The larger skin lesions from syphilis

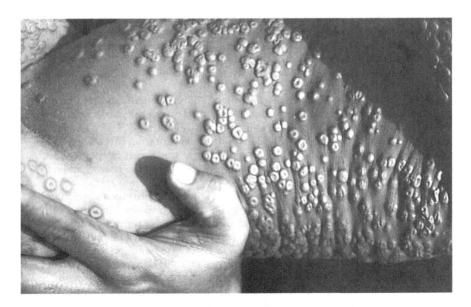

Figure 7.1 Smallpox skin lesions on the torso. If the picture was in color, the pustules would be surrounded by fiery red halos. This is best appreciated with the pox vesicles nearest the hand holding the child. (From Centers for Disease Control.)

DOI: 10.1201/9781003324058-7

were to be distinguished from the smaller ones of the ancient disease, now renamed *la petite verole* ("smallpox").

QUEEN ELIZABETH

Royalty and commoners were at equal risk. On October 10, 1562, the 29-year-old queen of England was at Hampton Court working on a letter to Mary Stuart. A missive designed to reconcile their differences. Later that day, Queen Elizabeth felt unwell and took a bath. She then went for a stroll among the autumn colors of her garden, hoping the stroll would shake off a minor disturbance to her constitution. It was a brisk day, and the queen began to chill.

Her doctors ordered her to bed, and to everyone's surprise, she followed their orders. She worked on what state papers she could, including the letter to Mary, but the fever mounted, and it became more difficult to concentrate. Elizabeth's advisors summoned the respected German-born physician, Dr. Burcot, to the palace. Although the queen's skin was still clear, he told her, "[M]y liege, thou shalt have the pox."

Frightened by the thought that she might have smallpox, Burcot's diagnosis angered the queen. Even if she survived, she stood an excellent chance of developing a scarred face. She cared about her life and appearance, more so since her rival, Mary Queen of Scots, was reputed to be beautiful. "Have away the knave out of my sight," she ordered. Insulted, Burcot went home.

Hours later, the queen became incoherent and sank into a coma. Even before then, Elizabeth and her advisors believed she was dying—unmarried and without a designated heir. Lords of the Privy Council were summoned from London and met in an adjoining room to discuss the question of succession. After the queen regained consciousness, she gave instructions to her waiting councillors.

They soothed her, promising to follow her instructions. But if she died now, England would suffer a religious civil war. The English reformation of Elizabeth's father, Henry VIII, would be in mortal peril. The worry was that the Catholic Mary in Scotland would attempt to reunite Scotland and England under her monarchy. Queen Elizabeth begged the council to appoint Lord Robert Dudley as the protector of the realm. She swore that "though she loved and had always loved Lord Robert dearly, nothing improper had ever passed between them."

Two men from the court were sent to fetch Dr. Burcot again and told him the queen was sick and wished his presence. Still upset from his earlier encounter, Burcot angrily replied, "By God's pestilence, will she be sick? There let her die! Call me a knave for my good will!" The faithful servant then threatened to cut out Dr. Burcot's heart on the spot if he did not help the queen. Speechless and furious, the doctor mounted his horse and galloped off to the palace, arriving well ahead of the queen's messengers.

"Almost too late, my liege," Burcot said as he entered the queen's bedchamber and saw her sweating body. He ordered a mattress to be placed in front of the fire. Then a scarlet flannel was wrapped around her like a mummy. Only her left hand protruded. The queen was placed near the fire. He gave her a drink from a small bottle. The heat seemed to draw red spots out on her exposed hand. "What is this, master doctor?" the frightened queen asked. "Tis the pox." Burcot replied.

Her fears confirmed, the young queen began to complain about how much she loathed the smallpox. In no mood for her complaints, Burcot asked her brusquely, "By God's pestilence, which is better, to have the pox in the hands, in the face, or in the heart and kill the whole body?"

The pustules did form on her body, but Elizabeth did not die. Much to the relief and surprise of her court, Elizabeth recovered gradually. By November 11, she could move to Somerset Palace. Soon she was writing Mary, Queen of Scots, again informing her that the disease had not left any scars on her face.

Unfortunately, the infection struck others in her court. Her nurse, Lady Mary Sydney, came down with smallpox, and the disease left her face disfigured. She was so scarred, she never appeared again at court without wearing a mask. Another nurse, Mrs. Pen, died of smallpox.

A grateful monarch gave Dr. Burcot 100 marks and a plot of land in Cornwall. Elizabeth was fortunate to survive. Yet, her heavy white makeup in later portraits likely covers smallpox scars. Elizabeth went on to rule and watch over England for another 41 years.[1]

THE VIRUS AND ITS DISEASE

The cause of smallpox is a virus named Variola major—a brick-shaped virus that can only be seen with electron microscopy. It is far too small to be seen with regular light microscopy. The difference between a virus and a bacterium is that a virus cannot replicate itself. A bacterium can reproduce. A virus has too few internal components to enable self-replication. It must invade a living host cell. After taking a cell hostage, the virus directs the cell to produce its own proteins, rather than the host's proteins. In a sense, the printing press of the cell changes to print the viral information, rather than its own template. These counterfeit proteins are reassembled into intact virions. Finally, the viral load becomes so high that the cell explodes (i.e., lyses) and the virions spread to contiguous cells. The incubation period from the time of exposure to the initial illness is 12 days, with little variation.

The onset of symptoms is unexpected. One minute, a person is walking about feeling healthy, and suddenly they are stricken down with a splitting headache and a knifing sensation in the back. Within 24 hours, they have chills and become feverish. The temperature often goes up to 104°F (or 40°C). Patients are often delirious or even comatose at this point.

On the third or fourth day of the attack, the symptoms abate. The temperature returns to normal, and the mental cloud seems to roll away. The victim looks and feels better, and unless he knows what the disease is, he may actually believe the worst is over. Alas, in the next 24 hours, they begin breaking out in a rash all over his skin. Sores appear on the face and forearms and spread to the upper arms and trunk. They congregate, particularly on the back. The sores go through changes to what doctors call macules, papules, vesicles, and finally, pustules. What this means is the sores appear first as red splotches. They then become palpable and raised, and then turn into blisters. By the time a sore matures, it is about 8 mm or a third of an inch in diameter. As the eruptions begin, the temperature spikes upward again, generally passing 103°F (39.4°C). Besides skin lesions, painful pox sores appear in the mouth and throat. The patient's voice is raspy and hoarse.

Some patients appear burned. Beyond the skin, which sometimes sloughs off, the virus can attack the lungs, heart, liver, intestines, and other internal organs. Victims reek of a particularly sickening odor. It is an understatement to say that the patient is miserable. Victims start voicing a wish for death to relieve their agony.

In one out of a hundred patients, the virus causes ulcerations of the cornea, leading to permanent blindness of the affected eye. In the nineteenth century, smallpox accounted for as many as a third of the population who were blind in society.

If the patient survives, the pox lesions crust and fall off, often leaving a scar. Given its predilection for the face, some victims suffered a permanent pockmarked face. Since the infection produces lifelong immunity, there were two advantages of facial scarring. One was the exemption from weeks-long quarantine[2] when the disease often ravaged the community. Two, some wives or husbands with scarring were also chosen because they would not die during a smallpox epidemic and leave the spouse alone to raise any remaining children.

Respiratory contamination usually spreads the virus. Most victims acquire the virus through droplet aerosol infection in the room or in the ventilation system, rather than face-to-face contact with a patient. The patient remains infectious from the onset of symptoms until the scabs fall off about 21 days later. Corpses of victims that died can be a significant source of virus. Sometimes clothing or blankets recently contaminated with pus or scabs can serve as vehicles for the virus, whereby victims that are not in direct contact with a patient can become infected.

Smallpox remained endemic in Europe throughout the Middle Ages. In the early eighteenth century, reports of an inoculation circulated. This method allegedly provided protection from future infection. Until this time, isolation and quarantine were the mainstays in the European defense against smallpox.

Before the eighteenth century, two schools of thought debated the cause of smallpox. The minority opinion held the miasmic theory, which attributed the disease to bad air. Most believed the disease was due to innate seeds present in every human being at birth. These seeds of disease seemed a natural extension of the humoral theory. As a result, copious bloodletting became the principal treatment.

Others recommended a drink prepared from sheep's dung for treating smallpox, the reason being that such a repugnant medicine would help drive out the occult influence. Miller describes a quarrel in London over the usefulness of purgatives in this condition. This culminated in a duel in the quadrangle of Gresham College.[3,4] What most authorities agreed upon was the observation that almost every person must have it once.

This distemper spares neither Age nor Sex; Rich and Poor are equally exposed to the Influence. What is the most unaccountable, and as wide from all other Fever, is that the Difference of Constitution is no preservative against its Attack; inasmuch, that few escape it, at one time or other.[5]

Such an observation lent logical support to the innate seed theory. But the results of inoculation pointed to a different direction.

INOCULATION

Lady Mary Wortley Montague popularized the idea of inoculation in England. An intelligent, strong-willed woman, Lady Mary was an early feminist. At 19, she eloped with Edward Wortley Montague, who was elected to Parliament three years later. In the year of the election, she caught smallpox, which left her without eyelashes and a pockmarked face. A year earlier, her 20-year-old brother had died of smallpox. Thus, when Edward Wortley Montague became Turkey's ambassador, his wife had a more than casual interest in the disease, despite not being a physician.

Two weeks after her arrival in Constantinople, she wrote her now famous letter, dated April 1, 1717, to her friend in London,

I will tell you a thing that will make you wish yourself here. The smallpox, so fatal, and so general amongst us, is here entirely harmless, by the invention of ingrafting, which is the term they give it. There is a set of old women who make it their business to perform the operation every autumn in September, when the great heat is abated. People send to one another to know if any of their family has a mind to have the smallpox. They make parties for this purpose. When they are met (commonly fifteen or sixteen together), the old woman comes with a nut-shell full of the matter of the best sort of smallpox and asks what vein you please to have opened. She immediately rips open that you offer her, with a large needle (which gives you no more pain than a common scratch) and puts into the vein, as much matter as can lie upon the head of her needle, and after that binds up the little wound with a hollow bit of shell. … The children or young patients play together all the rest of the day and are in perfect health to the eighth. Then the fever begins to seize them, and they keep their beds two days, rarely three. They have rarely above twenty or thirty in their faces, which never mark, and in eight days they are as well as before their illness. Where they are wounded, there remain running sores during the distemper, which I don't doubt is a great relief to it. Yearly thousands undergo this operation; and the French Ambassador says they take the smallpox here by way of diversion, as they take the waters in other countries. There is no example of anyone who had died in it: and you may believe I am well satisfied with the safety of this experiment, since I intend to try it on my dear little son. I am patriot enough to take pains to bring this useful invention into fashion in England, and I should not fail to write to some of our doctors very particularly about it.[6,7]

In March 1721, Lady Montague had her 5-year-old son inoculated. This was done by Charles Maitland, the embassy surgeon in Constantinople. After returning to London, she had Maitland inoculate her 4-year-old daughter in April 1721. This was the first professional inoculation in England.

Charles Maitland, who may also have helped enlist the interest of the royal family, was granted royal permission to conduct a trial. Six condemned prisoners were to be inoculated at Newgate Prison on August 9, 1721. The king's physicians witnessed this event with 25 other medical representatives, some of whom were members of the College of Physicians. The prisoners survived the inoculation, received their freedom, and one was later shown to be immune to smallpox by exposure to two children with the disease. The Prince of Wales's two daughters were then inoculated.

These royal inoculations began the firm establishment of inoculation as a standard medical procedure in England. However, the new practice was not immediately accepted on a wide scale. Fewer than 900 persons were inoculated in England and Scotland in the first eight years after inoculation was introduced. Many lay and medical persons were still unconvinced of its efficacy. The well-publicized deaths of the son of the Earl of Sunderland and of a footman of Lord Bathurst did not help. Both deaths occurred within a month of the royal inoculations and were publicly attributed to smallpox inoculation, although Hopkins believes this was incorrect.[8]

Another crucial factor in the retardation of inoculation was its exorbitant cost (10 guineas)[9] during the initial period. Inoculation was expensive due to the lengthy period of preparation. There was aftercare in special isolation houses. More costs involved bloodletting and purging, as well as the special medicines prescribed by attendant physicians. The cost included board and lodging during the five- or six-week period necessary for the whole operation.

Economics, though, soon dictated spreading the practice of inoculation. There are many examples of markets wrecked for more than a year because of the presence of smallpox. According to the local historian of Dartford in Kent, in 1741, "[T]he country people became so alarmed (about smallpox) that the market was nearly deserted and did not recover for some years."[10] Smallpox lurked in market towns for periods of up to two years in the pre-inoculation era. This could ruin the trade of a town for that period.

Market towns often suppressed public knowledge about smallpox. They would isolate smallpox cases in the local Pest House and keep quiet about it. According to Dimsdale, "[D]ue care is taken to bury the dead [from smallpox] privately."[11]

Financial considerations were of primary importance in determining the attitudes of parish authorities toward the inoculation of the poor. It was soon realized it was cheaper to inoculate the poor than to nurse, feed, isolate and sometimes bury them after they had caught natural smallpox. For example, the total expenditure of the parish of Castle Combe, Wiltshire, in 1758 due to a smallpox epidemic was £141. The parish could have inoculated its 560 people for £70, assuming each inoculation cost 2 shillings and sixpence per head. Since some were already immune, it is unlikely that the number needing inoculation was as high as 560. Not all poor would have to be paid for by the parish, as employers sometimes paid for the inoculation of their servants to minimize the danger to their own families.

That inoculation to prevent smallpox worked was undeniable to any reviewer. Mortality statistics from Boston show 700 deaths (out of a population of 4,000) due to the infection in 1677 prior to inoculation, for a rate of 175 deaths per thousand. With aggressive inoculation practices, deaths from smallpox fell to 284 (out of a population of 19,300) for a rate of 10 per thousand.

Why then were significant parts of the general population refusing inoculation? One reply could be that the population of the eighteenth century was largely uneducated and unable to appreciate statistical evidence. Resistance to inoculation came from more than the lack of appreciation for mathematical arguments. The principal opposition stemmed from the deadly side effect of live virus inoculation. Depending on technique, about one in a hundred of those inoculated died of the resulting infection—a horrific outcome when judged by modern standards. However, in the context of a 15%–90% mortality rate with universally acquired infection, the protection was obvious.

Second, the inoculees could spread the infection via the more dangerous route of respiratory secretions and pose a threat of recurrent epidemics to the community. Judging the results in a given village was not easy, as many municipalities forbade inoculation until an epidemic occurred, leading to the risk that many inoculated would have already been incubating the epidemically acquired virus before they had time to be protected. However, any subsequent deaths would always be blamed on the inoculation, not the epidemic. Even in these settings, the death rate for inoculees was still 5% or less. However, if a death occurred in one's own family, one might have a strong opinion about the practice.

Many, particularly in non-market towns, took the coward's approach. They held a vain hope that smallpox would not visit their town during their lifetime. Then they would not be exposed to the enormous risk of dying of natural smallpox or the small risk of dying of inoculation. Cowardly is the proper descriptor. The personal decision to avoid inoculation allows for an easier start to an epidemic. Immune persons form a social barrier (now referred to as herd immunity) against an infectious agent limited to humans.

The practice of inoculation appears to have been the primary reason for a greatly improved life expectancy during the eighteenth century. This would be the first time in history that life expectancy would actually improve.

Razzell records a comment from 1803:

One very great cause of increasing population may be ascribed to the success of inoculation for smallpox. One in four or five…usually died of this loathsome disorder in the natural way of infection….so that this saving of lives alone would account for our increasing number.[3]

GEORGE WASHINGTON

In the context of early American history, smallpox affected the struggle to win revolutionary Boston. After the battle of Bunker Hill in 1775, General Washington and the Continental army refused to attack British-occupied Boston for nine months. Refugees streaming into Boston apparently carried smallpox into the city. Most of General Howe's troops were immune from smallpox, as it was a long-standing policy for British soldiers to be inoculated.[12] In contrast, Washington's troops were much more susceptible since their countryside origins had not promoted inoculation. Washington, whose own pockmarked face attested to his survival from an attack in 1751, was afraid his uninoculated army might get infected.

From Cambridge, he wrote to Congress on July 21, 1775,

I have been particularly attentive to the least symptom of the smallpox: and hitherto we have been so fortunate to have every person removed, so soon as noting, to prevent any communication, but I am apprehensive it may gain in the camps. We shall continue the utmost vigilance against this most dangerous enemy.[8]

Washington suspected the British deliberately planted smallpox victims among the refugees they allowed to leave Boston. Washington had all refugees from Boston inspected and smoked to guard against contamination. On December 11, 1775, he wrote again to Congress,

The information I received that the Enemy intended to spread Smallpox among us I could not suppose them capable of. I now must give some credit to it, as it made its appearance on several of those who last came out of Boston. Every necessary precaution has been taken to prevent its being communicated to the Army.[8]

When the British did leave on March 17, Washington ordered 1,000 men who previously had smallpox to take possession of the city. Two days later, he was forced to send in most of his men to secure the needed supplies left by the British against the civilians that were pouring back into Boston.

One may conclude that the long nine-month deadlock between the American army and the British in Boston was due in a great degree to smallpox. The American commander did not want to be strategically hamstrung ever again from smallpox.

Orders were given in early 1777 to inoculate all soldiers who had not had smallpox. Many camps were set up in Virginia and elsewhere for the men to be treated and then recover for the extended time needed. This required absolute secrecy, or the enemy could overrun the camps.[8]

Due to Washington's astute judgment, most histories of the Revolutionary War do not even mention smallpox. Weaker leadership might have given a more chaotic outcome.

EDWARD JENNER AND VACCINATION

One of the most remarkable men in the history of medicine, Edward Jenner, MD (1749–1823), waded into the smallpox controversy in 1798. He published his 64-page treatise on preventing smallpox by vaccination with cowpox. This was different from inoculation with human smallpox.

Stimulated by a casual remark from a milkmaid in his practice, Sarah Nelmes, "I can't take the smallpox, for I've had cowpox." Jenner went on to transfer cowpox material on May 14, 1796, from Sarah's palm to the arm of 8-year-old James Phipps. The child developed a mild reaction to the inoculated cowpox a week later. This was like that after a favorable smallpox inoculation. On July 1, Jenner inoculated the boy with pus taken from a patient with smallpox. There was no significant reaction. The inoculation with the benign cowpox virus had made Phipps immune to smallpox. Jenner described his own reaction in a letter to a friend dated July 19, 1796:

> I was astonished at the close resemblance of the Pustules in some of their stages to the variolous Pustules. But now listen to the most delightful part of my story. The Boy has since been inoculated for the Smallpox, which as I ventured to predict produced no effect. I shall now pursue my Experiments with redoubled ardor.[13]

Jenner submitted a brief paper describing this single experiment about cowpox to the Royal Society in 1797. Because his evidence was so slim and his conclusion so audacious, the paper was returned. An appended note stated, "[I]f he valued his reputation already established by his paper on the cuckoo [see below], he had better not promulgate such ideas as the use of cowpox for the prevention of smallpox."

Not dissuaded, Jenner continued to vaccinate more cases, leading to his full-length report in 1798. (We have moved from calling an injection with cowpox "inoculation" to the word "vaccination." Vaccination [vacca meaning cow] indicates using animal-derived cowpox.)

What of Jenner's life before this? He received his medical degree from St. Andrew's College in Scotland in 1792, before returning to Berkeley, England. Jenner was the first to describe the unusual behavior of the cuckoo. This bird lays its eggs in other birds' nests. The foreign cuckoo hatchling then uses depressions on its back to eject the nest's rightful inhabitants. The non-cuckoo parents then raise their offspring's usurpers through some misplaced instinct. This natural history study of the cuckoo bird formed the basis of his election to the Royal Society in 1788.

It was well known in cattle-raising districts of England that an attack of cowpox made one resistant to smallpox inoculation. Jenner's unique contribution was not that he vaccinated a few persons with cowpox, but that he then proved they were immune to smallpox.[14] Moreover, he demonstrated that person-to-person inoculation of cowpox could occur. Cattle were not required. He receives credit by defending and proving the scientific merit of his technique.

The advantages of vaccination with cowpox versus inoculation with smallpox were obvious. It entailed no risk of spreading smallpox to the rest of the community. Vaccination was simpler and cheaper. Vaccinees did not need isolation for two or more weeks. Of most importance, deaths were rare from cowpox vaccination (one in a million).

A translation of Jenner's *Inquiry*[15] soon appeared in German, French, Spanish, Dutch, and Italian. In a short period, Jennerian vaccination supplanted inoculation around the world.

It was, as Edwardes writes, "as if an Angel's trumpet had sounded over the earth."[16]

BENEFITS AND OPPOSITION

Despite its manifest popularity and rapid utilization, vaccination was not embraced without opposition. Scientific, political, religious, and social objections soon arose. Scientific issues included controversy about the duration of immunity and its safety. While Jenner contended that vaccination, like the earlier inoculation, gave lifelong immunity. Yet, evidence accumulated by the 1830s that such was not always the case. Cases of smallpox could occur 20–30 years later. Yet, the disease was usually much milder and death rare. A second vaccination 10–20 years later was then often done for many patients.

The arm-to-arm vaccination was necessary for the early propagation of cowpox. This also transmitted other diseases, such as syphilis. In one episode at Rivalta, Italy, for example, 63 children were vaccinated with material taken from the pustule of a healthy infant. This infant had no external signs of infection with syphilis infection. Forty-four of the vaccinated infants developed overt syphilis. Several died of it, and some infected their mothers and nurses.

While solutions to these problems would be found, the difficulties supported opponents of vaccination. Opposition remained in the realm of health cults until compulsory vaccination. The benefits of vaccination were obvious. To do good to humanity was a function of the state, the medical profession, and the established church.

Vaccination was debated as an issue that balances the liberties of the individual against the community's well-being. Objectors were free riders who, reaping the benefits of herd immunity, themselves posed a threat to the community. Compulsion was therefore justified to ensure that all shared this common burden.

But for all its advantages, cowpox vaccination was in one respect more objectionable than inoculation. Vaccination required infecting humans with an animal virus. Some laymen could not believe that having one disease could protect against a different disease. The fact that cowpox came from animals enhanced their skepticism. Dixon notes others were understandably put on guard by rumors that cowpox was a venereal disease of cattle. Cartoonists depicted people that grew horns, tails, or acquired other bovine characteristics after being vaccinated. One woman complained after her daughter was vaccinated, she "coughed like a cow, and had grown hairy over her body"[10] (Figure 7.2).

Resistors were often firm believers in evolution, convinced that vaccination caused intimate biological contact between humans and lower forms of life. This counteracted progress of the species. In the most extreme formulations, the fear of species transgression led to prophecies of general decline from a countering of the laws of evolution.

One opponent went so far as to state that vaccination was the cause of masturbation, hysteria, sexual perversion, hemorrhoids, and a groaning smorgasbord of other ailments.[17]

For some, vaccination implied that the Creator had worked so imperfectly that his creatures were dangerous until punctured by a physician. A healthy, unvaccinated child was a threat to society, much like a mad dog or keg of gunpowder. "If God had wanted a vaccine injected into the blood, as one put it with a variant on the classic appeal to the obviousness of divine intention, he would have provided a suitable orifice."[12]

More typical were the actions of priests in Naples and Palermo, who led processions of people to be vaccinated. Some pastors not only were advocates

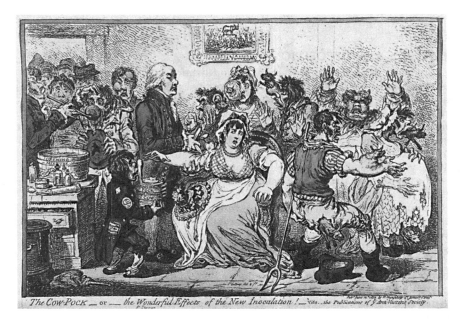

The Cow-Pock — or — the Wonderful Effects of the New Inoculation! — vide the Publications of ye Anti-Vaccine Society.

Figure 7.2 The Cow Pock. An 1802 British satiric cartoon showing the development of bovine features in vaccine recipients. (From Wellcome Library, London, CC Public Domain Mark 1.0.)

but actually vaccinated people themselves. Reverend Finch in Lancashire reportedly vaccinated more than 3,000 persons. Parents bringing their children for baptism in Geneva received literature promoting vaccination. During an epidemic in Rome in 1814, the Pope endorsed vaccination as "a precious discovery."[18]

Yet, forced vaccination drew ire from many. Once the state's right to wield the lancet had been admitted, one wondered where things would end. "Are we to be leeched, bled, blistered, burned, douched, frozen, pilled, potioned, lotioned by Act of Parliament?"[19] Some felt vaccination was medical terrorism inflicted by fanatics that happened to enjoy the backing of the state.[20]

On the other side, one observer succinctly stated, "Each French citizen has the right to die of smallpox, but he does not have the right to infect his fellow citizens."[21]

With exceptions, direct force was rare. The leverage available to the authorities consisted of fines and possible jail sentences. Fines ensured compliance almost as well as direct compulsion. With prosecution or accumulation of fines, the recalcitrant faced bankruptcy or jail. Objectors could choose to vaccinate their children or take the drastic punishment.

It is likely that repeated prosecutions for non-vaccination violated the legal principle of double jeopardy. That is, one cannot be punished twice for the same crime. Many prosecutions became the primary legal issue in the battle over compulsory vaccination in the nineteenth century. When the authorities in several nations eventually lost the opportunity to prosecute repeatedly, resistors could buy exemption from vaccination through payment of fines. Then the system became in effect voluntary.

Anti-vaccinators did not wish the state to take no action. Instead, they preferred an approach called neo-quarantinism. This tactic involved case reporting to the authorities, two weeks isolation, surveillance of contacts, disinfection, and even sometimes destruction of belongings and dwellings.[22] It would have been difficult to prove that neo-quarantinism worked, but in any case, no attempt to test the practice was offered. Isolation of smallpox victims had been undertaken in the past, but the fiery disease was still sweeping through the world. Still, pro-vaccinators argued the state had a right to restrict individual liberties for the common good. Vaccination (a quick jab twice a lifetime) was a less intrusive imposition than neo-quarantinism.[23]

Pro-vaccinators admitted that personal liberties were being abridged. Yet, this abridgment was no more intrusive than what Western societies were already doing with compulsory schooling, military service, and registration of births and deaths. Any line drawn at compulsory vaccination was thus arbitrary and capricious.[24]

Only a few years after his discovery, Jenner with remarkable insight predicted that "the annihilation of smallpox—the most dreadful scourge of the human race—will be the final result of this practice." The prevention of blindness alone in this condition "would suffice to render Jenner's name immortal."[25]

THE DEMISE OF SMALLPOX

We now fast-forward to the twentieth century. The conquest of smallpox marched on, as cases decreased to an annual rate of 110,000 in the United States in 1929. Then, it disappeared after 1949.

One of the last remarkable outbreaks occurred in New York City in March 1947. A businessman traveled by bus from Mexico to New York City, where he was hospitalized with a rash and fever. He died five days later. Two weeks after his death, smallpox was diagnosed. By that time, he had infected 4 people, who in turn infected 7 more, resulting in 12 cases and 2 deaths. The outbreak triggered near hysteria, with daily banner headlines in New York City. Municipal workers, with the fire department providing yeoman manpower, led to the emergency vaccination of more than six million people in less than a month (five million in less than two weeks). However, as expected (see the following), six vaccinees died of adverse reactions to the injection.[26]

Smallpox continued to decline in developed countries but persisted in undeveloped countries. In 1958, the World Health Organization (WHO) was asked to investigate the challenges of a global program to eliminate smallpox. The program languished until 1966, when the United States, the Soviet Union, and Sweden finally contributed large financial resources to a remarkable program of Cold War cooperation.

Yet, many doubted the possibility of successfully undertaking a coordinated global effort. One that would involve more than 50 developing countries, some of whom were among the poorest.

In 1967, 33 countries had endemic smallpox, and 14 others reported importations. The total population of the endemic countries was more than 1.2 billion. Most were developing countries in the tropics. Surveillance systems there identified perhaps 1% of the actual number of cases. Although 131,000 cases of smallpox were reported in 1967, as many as 10 to 15 million cases may have occurred that year.

Early on, there was debate on the best strategy to attack smallpox. Many felt that mass vaccination of everyone in endemic countries was necessary. Yet, malaria eradication had faltered with such a principle in the vast spaces of the Amazon in Brazil. Still, China had eliminated smallpox in 1960 after compulsory vaccination. However, few countries could match the dictatorial approach of the Chinese. The number of people needing vaccination in India and the isolated stretches of the Sahara sobered many planners.

As time went on, smallpox cases persisted in undeveloped countries, even when a 90% vaccination rate was achieved. Because of this, a strategy referred to as surveillance and containment was started. In what may be the most important publication in the campaign against smallpox since Jenner's monograph, Foege, Miller, and Lane published the technique in the 1972 issue of the *American Journal of Epidemiology*.[27] Briefly, the strategy involves identifying smallpox cases and vaccinating everyone within a five-kilometer radius and then searching for any other cases in an extra five-kilometer radius.

To encourage the reporting of possible smallpox cases, a special reward of $1,000 was offered. This would be given to the person and health-care worker that reported a possible case of smallpox, later confirmed. Tens of thousands of suspected cases were thus reported and investigated. Undoubtedly, the financial bounty (which exceeded the annual per capita income in most of these countries) was helpful.

A combination of mass vaccination and the surveillance method began to eliminate smallpox. The Americas became free of smallpox in 1972 when the last case in Brazil was recorded. In 1975, Asia recorded its last case in Bangladesh. The last case of natural smallpox in the world occurred in Somalia in October 1977, when a 23-year-old cook came down with the characteristic rash.[28] The WHO wanted to wait two years to check for any additional cases. None occurred. On December 9, 1979, the WHO produced an epic announcement, "Smallpox eradication has been achieved throughout the world!"

The most dreaded disease died.

BIOTERRORISM

Many have worried about the possible use of smallpox for bioterror purposes. The source would be from laboratory stocks. There are two WHO-sanctioned collections at the Centers for Disease Control and in Russia. But who knows if there are other hidden stocks? Smallpox could be devastating in a population with little residual immunity. Vaccination with smallpox stopped after 1983. People in the United States born after 1983 have no immunity. Moreover, the immunity of those vaccinated before 1983 is either partial or nonexistent.

Smallpox would be a very inefficient agent, as the disease is easily diagnosed by its rash. Secondary cases can easily be interdicted due to its lengthy 12-day incubation period. An intensive, selective containment and vaccination program initiated immediately after diagnosis should prevent all but a handful of cases in a third generation. This would stop the spread of the virus within four to six weeks.

The existence of possible terrorist use emphasizes the need for the security of laboratories holding Variola virus stocks. This security has been done in detail with periodic inspections of the two official WHO sites in Atlanta and Russia. Vaccine reserves will need to be maintained, along with expertise for diagnosis and control. The remote risk of a terrorist attack does not constitute a basis for the continued vaccination of the general public.

CONCLUSION

For the first time in the history of medicine, claims for and against a therapy involved mathematical arguments. Proof of preventing smallpox was developed in the battle for acceptance of inoculation. The tolerance of a 1%–2% mortality from inoculating smallpox highlights how fearsome the death rate from the universal infection was. This dilemma brings to light what is now called benefit risk. The latter numbers show the benefit of prevention and the cost of that prevention. Improved methods with smallpox vaccination still bring a one-in-a-million risk of neurological damage. When the likelihood of acquiring smallpox diminishes to near zero, then the risk-benefit ratio of the vaccine is no longer in favor of routine administration.

The eradication of smallpox was a milestone in the history of scientific medicine and international cooperation. For the first time, human beings set out to eradicate a universal disease and succeeded. A potential fate that could befall other vaccine-preventable infections, like polio, measles, or hepatitis B.

NOTES

1 Hopkins DR. *The Greatest Killer: Smallpox in History*. Chicago: University of Chicago Press; 2002, pp. 1–3.

2 From the Italian word *quarantos* meaning the 40-day wait the Venetians required of all foreign ships in the harbor before goods would be unloaded.

3 Ibid, p. 32.

4 An odd way of proving evidence in medicine—by dueling!

5 Razzell PE. Population change in eighteenth-century England. A reinterpretation. *Economic History Review* 1965;18; pp. 312–32.

6 Montagu LMW. *Embassy to Constantinople: The Travels of Lady Mary Wortley Montagu*. Amsterdam: Vintage; 1988, p. 121.

7 Typical of the promoter of any new treatment, Montague underestimates the toxicity of the therapy. Recipients of the direct virus method undoubtedly died at a 1% rate, but their deaths could often be ascribed to something else.

8 Hopkins, pp. 48–49.

9 It is difficult to gauge the value of a guinea. The value of labor varies by year, location, and occupation. A guinea was 21 shillings, or slightly more than a British pound. A guinea was about three days, wages for an agricultural laborer at the time. A guinea was the charge for a doctor's visit for the well-to-do.

10 Dunkin J. *The History and Antiquities of Dartford, with Topographical Notices of the Neighborhood*. Dartford, England: Palala Press; 1844, p. 398.

11 Dimsdale T. Tracts, on inoculation, written and published at St. Petersburg in the year 1768, by command of Her Imperial Majesty, the Empress of all Russia: with additional observations on epidemic small-pox, on the nature of that disease, and on the different success of the various modes of inoculation 1781. https://archive.org/details/b21441406 (accessed August 7, 2018).

12 Fenn EA. *Pox Americana: The Great Smallpox Epidemic of 1775–82*. New York: Macmillan; 2001, pp. 46–94.

13 Baron J. *The Life of Edward Jenner...With Illustrations of His Doctrines, and Selections from His Correspondence.* Cambridge: H. Colburn; 1827, p. 138.

14 Hopkins, p. 80.

15 Complete title—*An Inquiry into the Causes and Effects of the Variolæ Vaccine, or Cow-Pox. 1798.*

16 Hopkins, p. 79.

17 Baldwin P. *Contagion and the State in Europe, 1830–1930.* Cambridge: Cambridge University Press; 1999, pp. 283–4.

18 Hopkins, p. 83.

19 Gibbs J. *Reviews of Letters from Graefenberg, 1847–1854.* Gibbs, John, of Camberwell. Internet Archive. https://archive.org/details/b28748438 (accessed August 9, 2018).

20 Baldwin, p. 276.

21 Baldwin, p. 327.

22 How invasive is destruction of belongings and dwellings by the state compared to vaccination!

23 The reason quarantine did not work (and does not work for most infectious diseases) is that people are asymptomatic carriers, who can pass the infection, before they become ill.

24 Baldwin, p. 328.

25 Hopkins, p. 80.

26 Leavitt J. "Be Safe. Be Sure." New York City's Experience with Epidemic Smallpox. Chapter in: Rosner D, ed. *Hives of Sickness: Public Health and Epidemics in New York City.* New Jersey: Rutgers University Press; 1995: pp. 95–114.

27 Foege WH, Millar JD, Lane JM. Selective epidemiologic control in smallpox eradication. *American Journal of Epidemiology* 1971;94; pp. 311–5.

28 It should be noted that the position of anti-vaccinators that the disappearance of smallpox coincidentally occurred from improved sanitation and standard of living is absurd since the poorest countries where smallpox was cornered and eliminated had none of these advantages; the last countries involved were fortunate that the world swooped in with ring vaccination.

8 Antony Van Leeuwenhoek and the Microscope

No family, no fortune, no university degree. One would not have predicted scientific greatness from Antony Van Leeuwenhoek (pronounced "layu-wen-hook"). Born in 1632 in Delft, Holland, to a family of tradesmen, he spoke only Dutch. Despite abundant lifetime correspondence, Leeuwenhoek wrote little about his private life. By day, he was a cloth merchant and haberdasher. By night, with an endless curiosity, and a mind free from the scientific dogma of his day, Leeuwenhoek discovered bacteria, protozoa, and nearly started microbiology single-handedly. It was as if he entered Narnia through the wardrobe each time.[1]

A respected citizen of Delft, he was appointed in 1660 as chamberlain of the Worshipful Sheriffs of Delft. In 1669, after passing the examination, he was admitted to the profession of surveyor. In 1676, he was appointed executor of the insolvent estate of the famous painter, Jan Vermeer.[2]

The center of Delft has changed little from the way Leeuwenhoek knew it four centuries ago. The Old Church (1246) and the New Church (1510) are near the spacious market square, along with the fish and meat markets. Finally, the town hall (1620) can be viewed where Leeuwenhoek surely spent much time performing his civic duties.

Of the five children born to him in two marriages, only one, Maria, survived childhood. When Leeuwenhoek was 34 years old, his second wife died. For the next 57 years, the only family member to live with him was his faithful daughter, Maria, who never married.

It is unclear why or when Antony began to construct his microscopes. He must have been familiar with using simple magnifying glasses to inspect the quality of cloth. Leeuwenhoek's name reached international awareness when the well-known Delft physician

Reinier de Graaf[3] introduced him to the Royal Society in a letter dated April 28, 1673,

> I am writing to tell you that a certain most ingenious person here, named Leeuwenhoek, has devised microscopes which far surpass those which we have hitherto known...the enclosed letter from him, wherein he describes certain things which he has observed more accurately than previous authors, will afford you a sample of his work...and [he] is ready to receive tasks for more, if the Curious shall please to send him such.[4]

The Royal Society was a young organization that received its royal charter only 11 years earlier in 1662. The society was to recruit as many important correspondents abroad as possible, with the only qualifications being "no extraordinary preparations of learning; to have sound senses and truth is with them a sufficient qualification."[5,6]

Leeuwenhoek's first letter was requested by the Royal Society and sent. Contained in his first letter were observations on the mouthparts, sting, and eye of the bee. Since Robert Hooke, a member of the Royal Society, had described these bee parts a few years earlier, Leeuwenhoek's letter was not earthshaking. Leeuwenhoek must have had knowledge of Hooke's work, as he prepared his specimens in the same way.

Several years before, Hooke and others had constructed compound microscopes (i.e., microscopes with more than one lens). However, due to technical difficulties (image distortion) with the lenses, these early compound microscopes could not magnify objects more than 20 or 30 times the natural size.

DOI: 10.1201/9781003324058-8

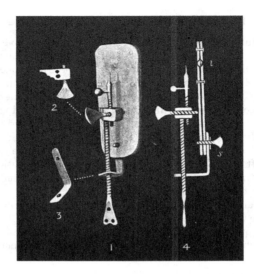

Figure 8.1 Leeuwenhoek's hand microscope. The symbol "[uncrossed t]" was the tiny convex lens. The specimen was put on the top of the needle in front (left of t). Vertical movement for focus was done thru screw 4. Horizontal movement screw 2. (Public Domain, Dobell Publications.)

Leeuwenhoek, on the other hand, used a simple, single-lens microscope. However, due to his skill in grinding lenses, he was able to construct an apparatus that magnified an object over 200 times (Figure 8.1).

One of the Dutchman's few surviving microscopes has been tested and found to have an astonishing (for the time) magnifying power of 300 times. As a result, his microscopes could distinguish far smaller objects than anyone else in the world.

Furthermore, Leeuwenhoek was the first microscopist to make ingenious calculations of the size of his objects. He first estimated the size of the human red blood cell to be 8 microns (a micron is a thousandth of a millimeter). Today, it has been measured at 7.2 microns.[7] His unusual precision is due to the fact that he was also an official land surveyor.

Leeuwenhoek's most famous letter to the Royal Society was his 18th letter dated October 9, 1676, and covers 17 large folio pages. In it, he recounts experiments from his diary as early as September 1675. The following selection is given to the reader, so they might obtain a flavor of his letters,

> I also discovered a second sort of animalcules, whose figure was an oval; and I imagine that their head was placed at the pointed end. These were a little bit bigger than the animalcules first mentioned. Their belly is flat, provided with divers [diverse] incredibly thin little feet, or little legs [i.e., cilia], which were moved very nimbly, and which I was able to discover only after sundry earnest efforts, and wherewith they brought off incredibly quick motions. ... These little animals would change their body into a perfectly round, but mostly when they came to lie high and dry. Their body was very yielding: for if they so much as brushed against a tiny filament, their body bent in, which bend also presently sprang out again; just as if you stuck your finger into a bladder full of water, and then, on removing the finger, the inpitting went away. Yet the greatest marvel was when I brought any of the

animalcules on a dry place, for then I saw them change themselves at last into a round, and then the upper part of the body rose up pyramid-like, with a point jutting out in the middle; and after thus lain moving their feet for a little while, they burst asunder, and the globules and a watery humor flowed away on all sides.[8,9]

Leeuwenhoek described three types of protozoa in the first part of his letter. In the next section, dated April 24, 1676, Leeuwenhoek states,

The fourth sort of creatures, which moved through the three former sorts, were incredibly small, and so small in my eye, that I judged, that if a hundred of them lay stretched out one by another, they would not equal the length of a coarse grain of sand; and according to this estimate, ten hundred thousand of them could not equal the dimensions of a grain of such coarse sand.[4]

His measurements indicated two to three microns, leaving no doubt he is describing bacteria for the first time. The Dutch microbiologist Kluyver says, "[T]here is every reason to consider the April 24, 1676, as the birthday of bacteriology."[10]

However, Leeuwenhoek's observations could not be verified with the inferior microscopes of the Royal Society. From April until November 1677, the Royal Society struggled in vain to repeat Leeuwenhoek's experiments. Finally, on November 15, Mr. Hooke succeeded in demonstrating the little animals so "exceedingly small that millions and millions might be contained in one drop of water." So many fellows observed them that there was no doubt of Leeuwenhoek's discovery.

Hooke also wrote Leeuwenhoek that King Charles II (founder of the Royal Society) was pleased with the demonstration of the little creatures (soon dubbed "animalcules") and "mentioned (with respect) your name simultaneously." This pleased Leeuwenhoek.[11]

After this, Leeuwenhoek's name was on the lips of everyone in the scientific world and high society. Nevertheless, it was a surprise to the unlettered Leeuwenhoek when he was unanimously offered a fellowship of the Royal Society in 1680, the highest honor one could then receive in the scientific world.

Upon receiving the certificate, which was worded in Dutch for his benefit, he wrote to Robert Hooke (who had given encouragement to the appointment), that he,

contemplated the document with great affection and my heart filled with gratitude; and with respect to you, Sir, I am bounden to say that not only this day, but all the days of my life, I am and will remain, Sir, with great thankfulness, your most obliged, Antony Leeuwenhoek.[12]

Leeuwenhoek evinces a deep religious assurance, a faith in the "All-wise Creator," and admiration for the perfection of the most minute, hidden mysteries of the work of his hands. He had a conviction that his research would help make "His Omnipotence" more universally known.[13]

Leeuwenhoek demonstrated the theoretical capillaries (connecting arteries and veins) predicted by William Harvey. These were noted in his 65th letter:

We see clearly with our eyes that the passing of blood from the arteries to the veins, in tadpoles, only takes place in such blood vessels as are so thin that only one corpuscle can be driven through at one time.

Leeuwenhoek continued a prolific correspondence and sent more information to the society than any other member in its venerated history. Of the 280 letters still in existence, most are to the Royal Society. Even on the day before his death, at age 91, he still dictated observations to the society (Figure 8.2).

While Leeuwenhoek never visited London after his election, the world came to him in Delft—Queen, Mary of England, and the Czar Peter the Great, both of whom he gave one of his microscopes. The visitors thronged so that he sometimes had to turn them away. Many of the fellows of the Royal Society came to Delft to witness firsthand the Dutchman's observations.

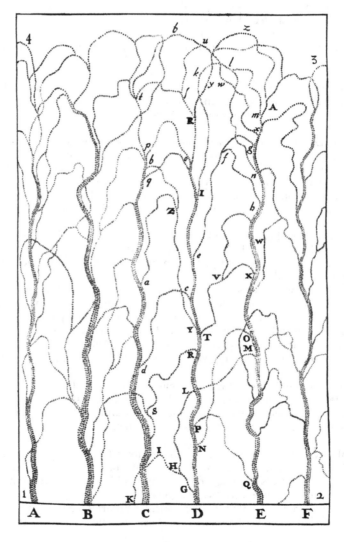

Figure 8.2 Leeuwenhoek's blood capillaries. The movement of blood from arteries to veins is demonstrated in the thin arcades at the top of the drawing. (From Wikipedia Commons.)

At the time, Leeuwenhoek was the only earnest microscopist in the world. The excellence of his lenses, combined with the exceptional keenness of his eye, surpassed all competition.

In 1981, British scientist Brian Ford discovered nine packets of biological specimens among the letters of Leeuwenhoek at the Royal Society in London. Ford published his examination of the surviving material through modern photography and demonstrates by comparison how well the drawings of Leeuwenhoek were done.[14]

Leeuwenhoek constructed over 500 microscopes during his lifetime but kept his manufacturing process secret. He gave few away but donated 26 of them to the Royal Society upon his death, where they remained for 100 years and then mysteriously disappeared. Only nine are now known to exist in museums around the world.

Leeuwenhoek's legacy is substantial. He opened the world of the unseen and revealed the presence of animalcules—organisms never discovered before. He was also the first to identify and measure red blood cells and human sperm.

Some have criticized Leeuwenhoek for not making the connection between his bacteria and disease. This is unfounded. Leeuwenhoek was not a physician. Furthermore, most laymen fail to realize that most bacteria and microbes are either helpful or benign to mankind. Therefore, it is difficult to pick out the malevolent ones.

Brian Ford argues Leeuwenhoek's approach described microbes within their milieu. He said, "Leeuwenhoek was closer to a true appreciation of their role in global ecology than much of contemporary science."[15] In any case, it took nearly a century and a half before the connection between microbes and disease was made with certainty by Pasteur and Koch.

In closing, two separate quotes from Leeuwenhoek are worthwhile:

My work, which I've done for a long time, was not pursued in order to gain the praise I now enjoy, but chiefly from a craving for knowledge, which I notice resides in me more than most other men. And therewith, whenever I found out anything remarkable, I have considered it my duty to put down my discovery on paper, so that all ingenious people could be informed thereof.

(June 12, 1716)

As I aim at nothing but Truth, and, so far as in me lieth, to point out mistakes that may have crept into certain matters. I hope that in so doing those I chance to censure will not take it ill. If they expose any errors in my own Discoveries, I'd esteem it as a Service; all the more, because it would thereby encourage me towards a nicer Accuracy.[16]

(December 25, 1700)

A thirst for knowledge and truth form the nucleus of any worthwhile scientist.

NOTES

1 See C.S. Lewis's *Chronicles of Narnia*.

2 Schierbeek A. *Measuring the Invisible World: The Life and Works of Antoni van Leeuwenhoek*. New York: Abelard-Schuman; 1959, p. 19.

3 The follicle in the human egg is still named the "Graafian follicle" after this physician who discovered it.

4 Dobell C. *Antony van Leeuwenhoek and His "Little Animals." Being Some Account of the Father of Protozoology and Bacteriology and His Multifarious Discoveries in These.* New York: Harcourt, Brace and Company, 1932.

5 Disciplines...Dover Publications reprint 1960 of 1932 edition by Russell and Russell; 1932, pp. 328–9.

6 Schierbeck, p. 29.

7 Schierbeek, p. 57.

8 Leeuwenhoek AV. *Concerning Little Animals Observed...in Rain-Well-Sea-and Snow Water.* London: Philosophical Transactions of the Royal Society of London; 1677.

9 This account clearly shows his observation of protozoa. His wonder at what we now call protoplasm without any skeletal parts or skin was an extreme novelty, as tiny animals were thought to be in structure like large animals only smaller.

10 Schierbeek, p. 65.

11 Schierbeek, p. 69.

12 Schierbeek, p. 34.

13 Schierbeek, p. 31.

14 Ford B. *The Leeuwenhoek Legacy.* London: Biopress and Farrand Press; 1993.

15 Ford B. Hidden Secrets in the Royal Society Archive. http://www.brianjford.com/wav-spc.htm (accessed August 16, 2018).

16 Dobell, p. 387.

9 Louis Pasteur, Anthrax, and Rabies

The scientific endeavors of Louis Pasteur are unmatched in history. In chemistry, he uncovered the mirror image of compounds; in microbiology, he solved the secrets of fermentation and prolonged the shelf life of milk; in medicine, he developed the first vaccines for anthrax and rabies.

Born in Dole, France on December 27, 1822, Pasteur possessed passion and creativity in his quest to unravel the mysteries of life. His family background provided the force of personality. Louis' father, Jean Joseph Pasteur, had little education but was a proud veteran of the armies of Napoleon. Conscripted in 1811, Jean Joseph rose to the rank of sergeant-major as a member of the Third Regiment. His battle-worn regiment was to begin in 1811 with 8,000 men and end in 1814 with only 284. Along with many other survivors of his regiment, he was given the Legion of Honor.

Upon the abdication of Napoleon in April 1814, Jean Joseph returned to Franche-Comte to resume his humble trade of tanning hides. His patriotic pride in France was a teaching repeated many times as the young Louis grew. Eventually, Louis attended the College of Besancon, only 30 miles from home. Here we find Pasteur working diligently in all his subjects and without evidence of homesickness. His standing at Besancon reflected his solid work—two times he was second in his class and once he took first place in physics.

After graduation, the prestigious graduate school, École Normale, was open to him. However, his place in the examinations placed him 15th out of 22 candidates. As evidence of his desire to always do better, Louis decided not to enter the École Normale at that point and took another year of preparation at the Barbet Boarding School. During his year at Barbet's, Pasteur attended lectures on chemistry at the Sorbonne by the celebrated chemist Jean-Baptiste Dumas. Pasteur wrote,

> The lecture hall is huge, and always filled. One has to be there a half hour early to get a good seat, just like in the theater. Here too there is a lot of applause. There are always between six and seven hundred listeners.[1]

Pasteur set his heart on becoming a chemist and resolved to devote himself to research. Repeating his entrance examinations in 1843, he realized his ambition of entering the École Normal by placing fourth in the list of entrants.

At the École Normal, Pasteur worked diligently and, judging from his letters, paid little attention to current events, such as the publication of *The Three Musketeers* by Alexander Dumas in 1844 or the restoration of Notre Dame in 1845. These events seemed not to have reached his consciousness.

Graduating in 1846, he stayed at École Normal as a graduate assistant in chemistry to Professor Balard. Pasteur worked in Balard's laboratory until 1848, where he was to make a stunning discovery, even as a neophyte scientist. As Pasteur was in the midst of composing his first major report in the early months of 1848, the usually imperturbable Pasteur was distracted by the sounds of rioting in the Parisian streets. What could be more important in life than the re-establishment of the republic and the glories of the empire?

In patriotic fever, Pasteur declared,

> We learn noble and sublime lessons from the events that take place under our eyes. Why, I am turning into a warrior when I hear all the noise of fighting and rioting, and if it became necessary, I would fight with the greatest courage for the sacred cause of the Republic.[2]

DOI: 10.1201/9781003324058-9

Pasteur's assistance ends up as a financial sacrifice, as one day he crossed the Place du Pantheon in late April and noticed a crowd gathered around a patriotic altar where contributions were being solicited. Pasteur hastened home to gather his life savings, amounting to 150 francs, and returned to deposit it in the defense of liberty, equality, and fraternity. The revolution succeeded, and a republic replaced the monarchy headed by Napoleon's nephew, Napoleon III. Pasteur and his father could not have been happier.

IDENTICAL COMPOUNDS?

Pasteur's first professional scientific project was to clarify a fundamental problem in chemistry. A current puzzle in chemistry was the apparently identical chemical compounds tartaric acid and paratartaric acid. Both were products of fruit fermentation and had been known for a long time. The riddle was reported in 1844 by the German scientist, Eihardt Mitscherlich. The problem was that while they had the same number of atoms and the same crystalline structure, their solubility and effect on polarized light were much different. Pasteur puzzled over the matter. This question struck at the basis of what was asserted in chemistry at the time. The modern reader must understand what was at stake—if the substances had the identical atomic composition, yet different physical properties, then the notion of a chemical species had to be revised. How could tartaric acid and paratartaric acid affect light so differently?

With extensive training in physics and crystallography, Pasteur approached the problem more broadly than previous chemists had. Through a series of experiments, Pasteur demonstrated tartaric acid rotated polarized light to the right and paratartaric acid rotated polarized light to the left.

In the midst of the political revolution of 1848, as mentioned previously, Pasteur reported his findings on the solution to the puzzle to the Paris Academy of Sciences on May 15. The implications of his research were immediately grasped. And, when others repeated his experiments, his name quickly rose in the scientific world.

What was discovered?

He had explained the baffling issue of isomorphism. In a single stroke, he started the field of stereochemistry; that is, the molecules of tartaric acid have an asymmetrical form in three dimensions. The human hands provide a simple analogy. The right and left hands are identical in composition, but everyone knows that the glove for one hand cannot be placed on the opposite hand. In fact, isomers are labeled "R" for right or "L" for left.

Beyond chemistry, his discovery opened up biology. Pasteur was one of the first to apply his discovery when he showed that the taste of food has to do with the form of the molecular isomer. The molecules of ingested food affect differently the nerve endings of the taste buds, depending on whether they are right or left-handed isomers. Sweetness is perceived with one and little taste from the other. Biological molecules, such as vitamins, enzymes, or antibodies, for the most part, are right-handed, and their left-handed counterparts are inactive. Pasteur was further challenged by the transformation of tartaric acid into its left-handed isomer. After much difficulty, he reported in 1853 he had done so. For this discovery, he was awarded 1,500 francs by the Paris Pharmaceutical Society and the Red Ribbon of the Legion of Honor. Vallery-Radot, the biographer son-in-law of Pasteur, states, "He had won it, not in the same way his father had, but he deserved it as fully."[2]

As the tartaric acid problem was related to fermentation of wine, Pasteur was then drawn into numerous studies on the poorly understood phenomenon of the breakdown of alcohol into vinegar. Over the next 15 years, his studies and scientific stature had grown to the point where when the French wine-making industry suffered serious losses from uncontrollable deterioration of wine, Emperor Napoleon III personally asked Pasteur to do what he could to ameliorate the emergency.

Pasteur discovered particular organisms accounting for the fermentation of wine into vinegar ("acid wine" at the time). Skepticism was considerable since microbes were not accepted as the cause of the problem. Pasteur merely waved the disbelief aside and found a solution. After considerable experimentation, he found that heating wine to 55°C sufficed to kill all these troublesome microbes without affecting the flavor of the wine. In doing so, he increased the shelf life from a few weeks to many years.

Confirmation, experiments performed by others, soon proved the validity of Pasteur's method now referred to pasteurization. Extension of pasteurization to milk in the early twentieth century eliminated the vexing problem of transmission of tuberculosis through milk.

One can imagine the gratitude of a culture where ingestion of wine is a central and daily activity. To enormously prolong the useful shelf life of such a universal household product made Pasteur a national hero. In 1867, members of the Universal Exposition presented Pasteur with a grand prize for his services to the wine industry.

Pasteur's successful resolution of a national difficulty earned him recognition from his emperor. Pasteur was invited to the national palace where Napoleon III listened to the mysteries of life and looked through Pasteur's microscope.

Despite a stroke at age 46, which rendered his left hand useless for the remainder of his life, Pasteur continued to expound the elements of his ideas and work that would culminate in his paper published in 1879 titled "The Germ Theory and Its Application to Medicine and Surgery."

While Pasteur was not the first to conceive of germs as causing disease, he and his German competitor Robert Koch generally agreed on the principles of the theory.[3] And while they did not coordinate their efforts about the subject (nor did they even like each other), they were the first in history to promulgate the principle in a comprehensive manner. Paul Bert is credited with launching the famous Pasteurian slogan: "One disease, one germ, one vaccine."[4]

ANTHRAX

In early 1877, Pasteur began looking into the veterinary epidemic of anthrax at the request of the minister of agriculture. At the time, anthrax was one of the deadliest infections for domestic animals. Horses, cows, and sheep were attacked in varying degrees, and annual victims were counted in the hundreds of thousands in France alone. Farmers considered themselves lucky if losses amounted to no more than 1 in 20 animals. The calamity struck the farm without warning. Farmers blamed it on poisoned pastures. The cause was unknown, but since the carcasses seemed charred, external causes, such as too much sun or herbal poisoning, were postulated. Stagnant water, horseflies, or foul air were also suspected. The disease developed rapidly. Animals simply collapsed and died immediately.

Even in scientific circles, the cause of anthrax was debated. The French physician, Davaine, was the first to notice little rod-shaped microorganisms in anthrax blood in the early 1850s. In 1863, Davaine injected blood infected with the microorganisms into rabbits and watched them die in short order. Skeptics argued it was some constitutional element in the blood, not the bacterium. Robert Koch attempted to sidestep the objections by placing pieces of spleen from diseased animals into the bloodless environment of the aqueous humor of the eyes—doing so, he produced as severe a case of anthrax as when blood was used. Opponents still argued that something intrinsic to body tissue was responsible. It fell to Pasteur to prove the point.

Pasteur began culture experiments using sterile urine, in which the bacillus of anthrax grows well. A drop of infected blood was placed into the medium. The bacteria were soon teeming throughout the medium. Then a drop of this culture was placed into a new one and grown; this was done a third time. If the first dilution is 1 to 1,000, the second would be 1 to 1,000,000 (compared to the original), and the third would be 1 to 1,000,000,000. After 10 such transfers, the amount of original inoculate present would be so diluted that it would be like a drop in the ocean. However, Pasteur kept diluting and diluting until he had made 40 successive transfers. After such efforts, not a single atom of the original blood was left, yet a drop of this culture injected into a guinea pig caused anthrax. "Anthrax, therefore," said Pasteur, "is the disease [which comes from] the bacteridium."[5] Most opponents of the bacterial theory capitulated and agreed.

Pasteur transferred a process of weakening bacteria (known as attenuation), which enabled him to create a vaccine for chicken cholera into one involving anthrax. While seeking to do so, he encountered difficulties with spores of the anthrax.[6] A few spores would contaminate Pasteur's attenuated anthrax cultures, which would revive when given favorable conditions and kill the animal. After many experiments, it was found that anthrax grown at 42°C–43°C (107°F–109°F) did not form spores. Under such conditions, the bacteria would become progressively weaker and eventually die in 30 days. Inoculating guinea pigs with this attenuated bacterium produced mild effects but rendered the small animals immune to later injections of anthrax.

THE PUBLIC TRIAL OF THE ANTHRAX VACCINE

Pasteur's announcement generated excitement, but as extensive experiments on larger domestic animals had not been done, the general attitude was one of suspended judgment. M. Rossignol, one of the editors of *Veterinary Press* and a critic of the germ theory, challenged the validity of Pasteur's findings. A short time before Pasteur's announcement about the anthrax vaccine, Rossignol had written,

> Microbiology is now the fashion, it reigns as a sovereign; it is a doctrine which one must not discuss; one must accept it without objections, especially when its chief priest, the learned Pasteur, has pronounced the sacramental words, "I have spoken." The microbe alone is and shall be the characteristic of a disease; this is understood and agreed to; henceforth the theory of germs should take precedence over pure clinics; the microbe only is eternally true and Pasteur is its prophet.[5]

Rossignol challenged Pasteur to a public test of his vaccine. Once Pasteur agreed, Rossignol began an active fundraising campaign for the public experiment. The Society of French Farmers soon rose to sponsor the project and placed 60 sheep at Pasteur's disposal.

On April 28, 1881, an energetic Pasteur communicated the experimental protocol he intended to follow. On day one, 25 sheep were to receive the preliminary dose of vaccine, and this was to be repeated on day 12. On day 26, virulent bacteria were to be injected into the vaccinated sheep, and also into the 25 unvaccinated sheep. It was anticipated that the unprotected animals injected with virulent anthrax should be dead in two to three days. Ten animals served as controls and received neither vaccine nor bacterial injections. The public demonstration was to be done at Rossignol's farm in Pouilly-Le-Fort with round-the-clock security to ensure no one interfered. May 5, 1881, was the day chosen for the first vaccination. A crowd of farmers, scientists, and reporters gathered in the small village of Brie.

The atmosphere was more like a county fair than a stuffy experiment. The press played up the affair into national prestige. Besides, how often can you see a distinguished scientist outside his laboratory? Amid a vast crowd of onlookers, Pasteur supervised his assistants as they gave the first injections. He was not to return until the end of the experiment.

Rossignol wrote, "These experiments are solemn ones and should become memorable, if, as M. Pasteur affirms with so much conviction, they confirm all that he has already claimed."[7] The editor also felt he had entered a no-lose public relations bonanza. If the experiment failed, it would be he who had found the national hero Pasteur wanting. If it succeeded, the honor of having thought of this dramatic outdoor experiment would go to him.

Even though Pasteur had published his findings, they were not as consistent and firm in his mind as he would have liked. Nevertheless, outwardly, he projected confidence.

On May 31, the inoculation with virulent anthrax took place. On June 1, Pasteur received a telegram from Rossignol informing him that all unvaccinated animals appeared ill and three were dead. Yet, among the vaccinated, all was not well. Twenty-one were well, but three had mild manifestations and one appeared ill.

Pasteur was seized with doubt. He even berated an assistant for causing the failure of the experiment until his wife, Marie, intervened to calm him down. The results became clear the following day. All unvaccinated animals challenged with anthrax died. The 10 controls were healthy. All the vaccinated animals challenged with anthrax were alive. Pasteur's laboratory received the news, and "there were cordial embraces all around amidst the guinea pigs," wrote Marie.[8] Pasteur returned to Pouilly-Le-Fort amid acclamation of the crowd, who applauded him as he stood around the carcasses of the dead animals. The skeptical Rossignol pronounced the experiment a great success and changed the name of his farm to "Clos Pasteur."

Suddenly, the vaccinated ewe, which appeared ill on June 1, died on June 4. The enthusiasm ended, and opponents were hopeful. But an immediate autopsy left no doubt: the cause of death was not anthrax, but a miscarriage, for the animal was pregnant.

The jury commissioned for the affair concluded no further experiments were needed. The vaccine was effective. The worldwide press agreed. It had taken a century for the scientific world to produce a second proven vaccine, like the one for smallpox. Realistic hope soared that more vaccines against other diseases could be produced.

Demand for the vaccine was high, and by the end of 1883, over 500,000 animals were vaccinated. Millions of animals have been spared the brutal disease since then.

RABIES

In a comparable manner, Pasteur attacked the problem of rabies—a most dreadful disease. The images of enraged animals foaming at the mouth and howling, with bloodshot eyes, ready to savagely attack man or beast have always filled the popular imagination with fear. Animals suffered the most, but when bitten, the infection could be transmitted to man. The incubation period is at least two weeks, and often up to six weeks or more. The symptoms of the furious attack by rabies drew investigators' attention to the nervous system. We now know the virus grows slowly from the peripheral nerves up the nervous system until the brain is reached. At that time, severe muscle spasms seize the entire body for hours in an agonizing manner that culminates in death.

The traditional term for rabies was hydrophobia due to the belief that rabid animals were fearful of water. In a magical manner, threatened villagers would place buckets of water at every street corner, hoping to ward off infected animals. Eventually, the alleged water avoidance behavior of rabid animals was proven untrue.

Not all rabid animal bites result in transmission. The proportion of bite victims that develop the disease ranges from 16%–25%, a risk influenced by the number and severity of wounds inflicted. But if the infection develops, all victims die.

Beyond mortality, there is the psychological dread that rabies injects into the relations between pets and owners—the fear that arises when animals show any change of attitude or the "slight uneasiness we always feel at the caresses of the animal in which nature best shows us her benevolent smile."[9]

We might wonder why Pasteur chose rabies as a subject of research. After all, it was an uncommon disease with only a few hundred deaths a year in France.

It is possible a childhood nightmare was responsible. Pasteur was eight years old at the time a rabid wolf went on the rampage near his home, biting man and beast. He observed a group of men carrying a man, who had just been bitten by the horrible beast, into the blacksmith's house. The victim had multiple bites, which were covered by bloody slaver, cauterized with a red-hot iron. The boy Louis watched in horror. Eight victims died of the disease from this episode, and the terror of the rabid monster haunted the region, and perhaps Pasteur's mind, for a long time.

It seems likely to the author that Pasteur chose rabies since it was a human affliction that already had an animal model available for study.[10] For whatever reason, rabies is the disease most associated with Pasteur in the popular imagination.

While Pasteur used the term "virus" in describing the rabies agent, he did not employ it in the twentieth-first-century sense, but merely as a generic term for any infectious agent. The official definition for the category of virus came about ten years later. A virus was operationally defined as an infectious agent so small that it could be passed through a porcelain filter known to stop all bacterial agents and for which attempts at culturing on standard media were unsuccessful. It was not until 1963 that the electron microscope identified viral particles of rabies in brain tissue.

Pasteur reasoned that given the long incubation periods, the infection could be aborted by giving a weakened rabies virus with a shortened incubation period. But how could he obtain such an attenuated virus?

After many failed experiments, Pasteur's breakthrough came on a particular day as he watched his assistant, Dr. Roux, who had been working independently, string an infected rabbit's spinal cord between the arms of the flask. Struck by this ingenious device, Pasteur modified and enlarged the flask and added caustic potash to dry out the nerve tissue. After 14 days, the spinal cord had lost its virulence (i.e., the ability to cause rabies), but not its ability to stimulate immunity (a concept that Pasteur was the first to promote). If this material is injected into a test animal, nothing happens. The next day, a spinal cord dried for 13 days is injected, and this process is repeated for another ten days. Finally, Pasteur injected a spinal cord, dried for only two days. If instead, this 2-day-old preparation was injected into an untreated animal, there would be a 100% chance of death. Yet, with the 12 days of inoculation, the animal produced no signs of disease. When the immunization process was begun after a known rabies injection, the protection was also 100%—not a single animal died. Then, Pasteur and his associates showed that animals bitten by a rabid dog and treated with the attenuated material avoided death, while control animals usually died.

The manner in which to begin the inevitable human trials worried Pasteur. He even considered inoculating himself with rabies and then taking the injections for protection.

As Pasteur struggled over the ethics of human research, circumstances forced his hand. A mother brought her 9-year-old boy, Joseph Meister, to Pasteur's laboratory on July 6, 1885. Two days earlier, the boy went to school alone when he was ferociously attacked by a mad dog and thrown to the ground. Too small to defend himself, he covered his face with his hands. A nearby bricklayer rescued Joseph and shot the dog. He picked up the boy, who was severely bitten about the face and hands, and took him home. Examination of the dog by veterinarians left no doubt as to its rabid state. The town physician, Dr. Weber, was consulted. He washed and cauterized the 14 wounds. He advised the parents to take the boy to Paris for a consultation with Pasteur since the number of wounds and their location on the face made the case alarming.

As Pasteur was not a physician, he had Joseph examined by two well-respected physicians. Both urged him to begin the vaccinations since the boy had a significant probability of dying without intervention. Pasteur reluctantly accepted their advice and began the series of injections for 14 days.

Joseph took the injections well. While he was constantly monitored in the laboratory, the laboratory became a type of farm, where the country boy found the chickens and rabbits to which he was accustomed. The lad even enjoyed playing with the white mice.

As the inoculated matter became more virulent, Pasteur became uneasy. A complication or death with Joseph would set off a firestorm of political and scientific criticism. After the last injection, a 1-day-old rabid spinal cord, given on July 16, Marie Pasteur wrote to her children, "My dear children, this will be another bad night for your father. He cannot come to terms with the idea of applying a measure of last resort to this child. And yet now he has to go through with it. The little fellow continues to feel well."[11]

Normally, an experimental animal would have rabies seven days after the virulent 2-day-old spinal cord was administered, yet Joseph felt well on discharge July 27 (post-injection day 11) and upon follow-up. While Pasteur attempted to downplay the incident, the press seized upon his exploit and spread the news. Pasteur stayed in touch with Joseph through numerous letters. He took an interest in the boy's education and future, so much as to open a savings account to cover small expenses.

Pasteur's method succeeded in several more cases, but it did not perform miracles. A child of 10, Louise Pelletier, was brought to Pasteur on November 9, 1885, 37 days after her wounds were inflicted. The aging scientist hesitated. His scientific self-interest dictated he should refuse since the treatment would surely fail. But moved by the parents' pleas and the child's suffering, he reluctantly proceeded. The child died of convulsive spasms seven days later, after only seven of the attenuated injections were given.

Pasteur's adversaries sought to exploit the failure, but they were unable to shake the public's confidence. They would have been silenced if they had read a letter written years later to Pasteur's biographer, Vallery-Radot, by the father of Louise Pelletier:

Among the prominent men about whose life I have learned, none seems greater to me. I do not consider them capable, as he was in the case of our little girl, of sacrificing long years of work, of endangering a universal reputation as a scientist, and knowingly risking a painful failure, out of simple humanity.[12]

Pasteur's work was little known in the United States until December 1885, when four American children, the sons of workers at the port of Newark, were bitten by a rabid dog. Pasteur accepted their treatment by telegram on the condition they sail immediately for France. The *New York Herald Tribune* paid for their passage by means of a public subscription for the children. The four little Americans arrived in Paris—accompanied by a doctor and the mother of the youngest of them, a boy only 5 years old. After the first inoculation, this little boy, pleased over the small pinprick, exclaimed, "Is this all we have come such a long journey for?" For several weeks, their adventure made the front pages of the daily papers in the United States. The quartet had arrived in time for the treatments to work.

Upon their return, the cured children were enthusiastically received and displayed in a Bowery shop window in New York City, where 300,000 curiosity seekers paid to obtain a glimpse of the youngsters. In addition, the children were asked many questions about the distinguished man who had taken such care of them. Needless to say, this incident provided unexpected and wonderful publicity for Pasteur and his germ theory.

Several months of incessant newspaper coverage made the idea that the rabies vaccine was a "cure," though it was really a preventative. The months of publicity about the matter created a different expectation for medicine in the United States. "In the process, popular consciousness gained an entirely new idea that medical research could provide widespread benefits. This new expectation about progress helped displace a centuries-old understanding (shared by physicians and patients alike) that little ever changed in medicine."[13]

By March of the following year, in 1886, Pasteur was able to report to the Academy of Sciences that only one death had occurred in 350 cases, Louise Pelletier. In August, Pasteur responded to his persistent critics:

How difficult it is to obtain the triumph of truth! Opposition is a practical stimulant, but bad faith is a pitiable thing. How is it that they are not struck with the results as shown by statistics? From 1880 to 1885, 60 persons are stated to have died of hydrophobia in Paris hospitals. However, since November 1, 1885, when the prophylactic method was started in my laboratory, only three deaths have occurred in these hospitals, two of which were cases which had not been treated.[14]

In March 1886, a subscription was begun to create the Pasteur Institute. The scientist wished it built without government funds. The institute was needed to treat the overwhelming number of rabies victims streaming into Paris and to research other infectious diseases. On November 14, 1888, the research and treatment center opened to a large inauguration in the building's library, attended by a sizable retinue of politicians and scientists.

Included within the institute for Marie and Louis Pasteur were living quarters. Inside the apartment, there was a spacious reception area to entertain the multitude of visitors that came to see the eminent scientist.[15]

As with his work with wine, the proof of Pasteur's vaccine work consisted of numerical comparison. The contrast in mortality between the sheep vaccinated or not, and the humans bitten by rabid animals, is striking. Mortality is the best point of comparison since it is an unequivocal diagnosis.

Pasteur suffered a second stroke and then died on September 27, 1895—holding a crucifix in one hand and the other resting in the grasp of Madame Pasteur. An immense funeral procession moved from the Pasteur Institute to Notre Dame. The French government gave consent for Louis, and eventually Marie, to be buried in a chapel built in the cellar of the Institute, rather than in the Pantheon with other French heroes. Above his crypt are four angels watching over him: Faith, Hope, Charity, and Science. There, Pasteur is keeping watch over his laboratories where his work continues.

NOTES

1   Debre P. *Louis Pasteur*. Baltimore: Johns Hopkins University Press; 2000, p. 23.

2   Vallery-Radot R. *The Life of Pasteur*. New York: McClure, Phillips; 1902, Kindle book, p. 70.

3   Robert Koch was the discoverer of the tubercle bacterium, and as such, his story is contained in Chapter 12.

4   Debre, p. 369.

5   Holmes SJ. *Louis Pasteur*. New York: Dover Publications; 1924, p. 100.

6   Spores are a metabolically inactive form of the bacterium that are adapted for prolonged survival under adverse conditions, such as exposure to heat, drying, or freezing. This feature of anthrax remains a problem today by making it difficult to be certain that an area has been cleared of anthrax, such as the cleaning of the US Senate offices in 2001.

7   Adelaide H. *Modern Biography*. San Diego: Harcourt, Brace, 1926, p. 139.

8   Debre, p. 401.

9   Debre, p. 414.

10   Obtaining an animal model for a disease is usually the first and often most difficult aspect of studying a disease.

11   Debre, p. 440.

12   Debre, p. 445.

13   Hansen B. *Picturing Medical Progress from Pasteur to Polio: A History of Mass Media Images and Popular Attitudes in America*. New Brunswick, New Jersey: Rutgers University Press; 2009, p. 47.

14   Vallery-Radot, p. 432.

15   The Pasteur Museum in Paris is well worth a visit. Contact the museum ahead of time to be sure it is open. It was closed in March 2017, but they opened it by appointment.

10 Wilhelm Roentgen, X-rays, and Bullets

In 1862, a 17-year-old Prussian lad named Wilhelm Roentgen (Vil-helm Ren-ken) admired a caricature of an unpopular teacher drawn by a friend. The schoolmaster entered and demanded the name of the artist. Despite painful cross-examination by the schoolmaster, Wilhelm refused to name the fellow student and was expelled.

Such an incident reveals the integrity and stubbornness of our next scientist. This incident shaped his future since his expulsion prevented him from earning an Abitur (diploma) in any German gymnasium (i.e., high school). He thus matriculated in 1865 at the Polytechnic School in Zurich, Switzerland (which did not require an Abitur), where he earned a mechanical engineering degree. He also learned to construct intricate laboratory instruments.

It was Roentgen's exceptional skill in constructing instruments that attracted Dr. August Kundt, one of the best theoretical physicists in Europe. He urged Roentgen to become his assistant at the University of Zurich. Kundt also made it possible for the young man to study for his doctorate in physics. It was in Zurich that Roentgen met his future wife, Anna Bertha, six years older.

In 1872, he was firmly established as an assistant to Kundt, who had moved to the prestigious University of Würzburg. Roentgen, with doctorate in hand, decided to move with Kundt. The distance from Anna Bertha induced him to marry her. Described as "slender, reasonably attractive and fairly well educated," she was satisfied to be the wife of a physics professor. She did everything possible to keep household affairs from distracting her husband's research. From all accounts, Bertha and Wilhelm were a devoted couple.

In 1895, at age 50, Roentgen had risen to full professor of physics at the University of Würzburg, where he was in the midst of experiments with a Crookes tube (Figure 10.1).

Sir William Crookes, a contemporary and one of England's most distinguished physicists, studied the effects of electrical discharges on rare gases. His tube was constructed as a glass cylinder, where a pump evacuated air, creating a vacuum. The cylinder also contained positive and negative electrodes for the discharge of a high-voltage current between them. The passage of the current was affected by the emission of what came to be known as cathode rays. Cathode rays were well-known and eventually became understood as something we now call electrons.

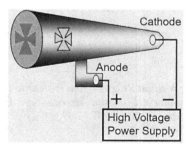

Figure 10.1 Diagram of a Crookes tube or cathode ray tube. The Maltese Cross was a piece of metal that blocked the passage of electron or cathode rays within the vacuum tube. This produced a shadow on the screen. Later in the twentieth century, early versions of computer or television screens were sophisticated cathode ray tubes. (From Wikimedia Commons.)

 DOI: 10.1201/9781003324058-10

However, other radiation was being emitted from the tube, which even the inventor had unknowingly witnessed. Crookes had stored unexposed photographic plates near his vacuum cylinder. Later, upon examining these plates, which were protected from light by wooden cassettes, he noted that some of them were flawed by shadows. Crooke went so far as to write to the manufacturer of the plates to complain they were damaged prior to his use.

Others had also encountered this effect, as scores of other Crookes tubes were in existence around the globe. What distinguished Roentgen, as with any great discoverer, was the pursuit and characterization of this strange phenomenon.

Repeating standard investigations with the tube in his dark laboratory, Roentgen noticed a greenish-yellow color flickering brightly about a yard from where he was standing. Startled by this eerie flashing, he at first thought he might have imagined the phenomenon. But when he again electrically excited the cardboard-covered tube, the flickering, flashing spurts of greenish yellow reappeared, only to disappear when the electric current was switched off. Mystified, he lit a match and peered at the site where the colors had appeared. He immediately spotted another screen coated with barium platinocyanide that he had left on his bench. Excitedly, he switched the current to the tube on and off, on and off. Each time he switched the current on, the screen began to fluoresce, explaining in part the strange burst of colors he had been observing.

Completely unsolved was the cause of fluorescence. It was clear that some sort of emanation was coming from the Crookes tube upon electrical excitement. But what was the nature of this discharge? Roentgen knew it could not be cathode rays—such rays cannot travel more than several inches in ordinary air, and the fluorescent screen when he first saw it glitter was a yard from the tube. Moreover, when Roentgen carried the screen from the bench to a new location many yards from the tube, it still fluoresced brightly when he electrically excited his tube. He sensed he might be producing a new type of electromagnetic wave.[1]

In succeeding weeks, Roentgen devoted himself to identifying more properties of the emanation. Weeks in which he ate and even slept in his laboratory. He found that a deck of cards or a two-inch thick book did not stop the fluorescence, but a thin sheet of lead stopped the rays completely.

To further test the ability of lead to stop the rays, he held a lead piece up to the aperture. To his amazement, he saw not only the shadow of the lead piece form but also that he could distinguish the outline of his thumb and finger (within which appeared darker shadows—the bones of his hand). Roentgen soon named these rays "X-rays," denoting them as from an unknown source.

In the midst of his many secret experiments defining the physical properties of X-rays over the next four weeks, Roentgen invited Mrs. Roentgen to his laboratory. He placed her hand on a cassette loaded with a photographic plate, upon which he directed rays from his tube for six minutes. On the developed plates (Figure 10.2), the dark shadows of her bones were clearly visible, along with the two rings on her finger. When he showed the picture to her, she shuddered at the thought that she was eyeing her own skeleton. To Bertha, as many others later, this experience gave a premonition of death; though this foreboding was not true, as Bertha lived another 24 years to die at age 80.

Once Wilhelm Roentgen was convinced of the soundness of his experimental observations, he drew his conclusions into a paper. The title was "On a New Kind of Ray: A Preliminary Communication," and he forwarded it to the secretary of the Würzburg Physical Medical Society on December 28, 1895. The report was published within a week. Knowing that publication in a local physics journal would not achieve worldwide recognition, Roentgen had reprints of his article made at his own expense and on New Year's Day sent reprints to six

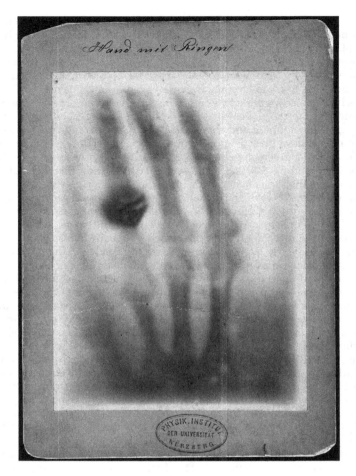

Figure 10.2 This is a photograph of a radiograph taken by Roentgen on December 22, 1896. It shows his wife's left bony hand where she is wearing a double ring.

of the most important physicists in Europe, along with the X-ray photographs of Bertha's hand. What prompted the immediate publication and focused the European physicists on Roentgen's work was not the factual description of his new discovery, but the X-ray picture of Bertha's hand.

One of the recipients of the reprint was Franz Exner, a physics professor in Vienna. Dr. Exner was so fascinated with the X-ray of the hand that he showed it at a party the next night—thereby both astonishing and terrifying the visitors. One of the guests relayed the information to the editor of Vienna's most prestigious paper, where a complete story was splashed across the Sunday, January 5, issue of *Die Presse*. In the following week, newspapers all over the world reported Roentgen's discovery.

A horde of scientists, reporters, and curious descended upon the modest institute at the University of Würzburg. "Our domestic peace is gone," complained

Mrs. Roentgen. Visitors went as far as to filch X-ray photographs from his laboratory, and postcards with Roentgen's signature failed to reach their destination.

The public recognized the value of Roentgen's discovery. A Frankfurt newspaper stated on January 7, 1896,

> We wish only to call attention to the importance this discovery would have in the diagnosis of diseases and injuries of bones, provided the process can be developed technically so that not only the human hand can be photographed, but also that details of other bones may be shown without the flesh. The surgeon then could determine the extent of a complicated bone fracture without the manual examination, which is so painful to the patient; he could find the position of a foreign body, such as a bullet or piece of shell, much more easily than possible heretofore and without any painful examinations with a probe. Such photographs also would be invaluable in diagnosing bone disease, which does not originate from an injury, and would help guide the way in therapy.[2]

Indeed, within six months, Roentgen's apparatus was being used to locate bullets by battlefield physicians in wounded soldiers. The immediate effect was that X-rays greatly reduced the number of amputations performed.

Not all understood the nature of the X-ray, dubbed by some as the "death ray." In London, a firm advertised the "sale of x-ray proof underclothing" in February 1896. A bill was soon introduced into the New Jersey state legislature to prohibit the use of X-rays in opera glasses.[3]

The list of honors Roentgen received is too long to enumerate. His recognition culminated with the Nobel Prize for Physics in 1901, the first year for this international award.

Though not rich by any means, Roentgen refused to gain from his discovery,

> According to the good tradition of German university professors, I believe their discoveries and inventions belong to humanity, and should not be hampered by patents, licenses, contracts, nor controlled by any one group.[4]

Thomas Edison felt otherwise:

> Professor Roentgen probably does not draw one dollar profit from his discovery. He belongs to those pure scientists who study for pleasure and love to delve into the secrets of nature. After they have discovered something wonderful, someone else must look at it from the commercial point of view. This will be the case with Roentgen's discovery. One must determine how to use it and to profit from it financially.[5]

Roentgen also donated the Nobel Prize money to his beloved University of Würzburg, the only scientist ever to do so with the Nobel award. Doing so led the Roentgens into extreme privation later during the harsh days of World War I and the postwar depression years in Germany.

Bertha required multiple daily shots of morphine during her last two years of life, and these were faithfully administered by her sanguine husband. Bertha died in 1919, and Wilhelm followed her in 1922.

Proof of Roentgen's discovery came from others that could easily reproduce his observations. Medicine was the first discipline to improve with the application of this newly discovered physical beam. Chest X-rays revolutionized the evaluation of tuberculosis (Chapter 12).

Friedman paid tribute:

No more honest or straightforward scientist than Wilhelm Conrad Roentgen ever lived. He literally had no discernible vices. He was a brilliant man, but his brilliance was tightly focused in that he lacked the conceptual grandeur of Isaac Newton or Albert Einstein. Still, when serendipity presented him with the flashing bit of fluorescing screen, Roentgen was not found wanting.[6]

NOTES

1 Friedman M. *Medicine's 10 Greatest Discoveries*. Oxford: Yale University Press; 1998, pp. 119–20.

2 Glasser O. *Wilhelm Conrad Röntgen and the Early History of the Roentgen Rays*. London: Norman Publications; 1993, p. 201.

3 Glasser O, Röntgen WC. WC Roentgen: Thomas; 1958, p. 82.

4 Glasser, Early History of the Roentgen Rays, p. 349.

5 Edison on Professor Roentgen's Discovery. Western Electrician. February 22, 1896. (This article cites the *New York Herald* as a source but does not give a date.)

6 Friedman, p. 130.

11 Ether, William Morton, and a Yankee Dodge

Pain. Pain. Pain. The concept of major surgery before the introduction of general anesthesia is incomprehensible to the modern reader. Cutting, pulling, and sewing flesh—maneuvers that have all been used as forms of torture. Before anesthesia, surgery was rushed and overly destructive. For below-knee amputations, instead of taking hours to trim each small structure (e.g., multiple arteries, veins, muscles) and create a covering skin flap, amputations were performed in seconds with a saw and the stump covered with hot tar. The greatest surgeons were the quickest—since blood loss and survival in the awake patient were best preserved with dispatch.

Attempts to ameliorate the horror of surgery before 1846 were ineffectual and dangerous. Different forms of narcotics have been known for over three millennia. The use of opium (extracted from the poppy plant) is described by most ancient civilizations that appreciated that the preparation induced sleep, relieved cough, and alleviated pain. Unfortunately, the oblivion that can be achieved with high-dose narcotics is often permanent. Alcohol is even worse for anesthesia than narcotics. While a large amount of alcohol can render one stuporous, it does little to mask pain. Alcohol in high doses depresses heart and lung function, and the fatal dose of alcohol, as for opiates, is not much higher than the coma-inducing dose. When alcohol and narcotics are combined, they are even more hazardous.

In some jurisdictions, the death of a patient from opiate and alcohol anesthesia was punishable by death for the doctor. As a result, both the patient and doctor preferred pain to death. Though in many instances, patients refused the torture of surgery and submitted to the alternative of impending disability or death. Instances of suicide before surgery were well known.

Surgeons were not unaffected. A humane person cannot inflict pain without sharing it in good measure. If they could not learn to harden themselves, they left the profession in droves, or often drank as much as the preoperative patient did.

While not wishing to further the readers' squeamishness, our modern attitude of taking general anesthesia for granted must be suspended to enter into the marvelous significance of this discovery. The controversial idea of producing painless surgery at the time of our next story was the practice of mesmerism. Available in England in the 1830s and 1840s, mesmerism was performed in a few other places. It is difficult to know exactly what was involved with the technique of mesmerizing in the mid-nineteenth century. The modern reader can substitute the more recent practice of hypnosis as an approximate equivalent.[1]

NITROUS OXIDE AND ETHER

In 1844, Horace Wells, a 29-year-old dentist in Connecticut, attended a demonstration by an itinerant lecturer on nitrous oxide. The so-called laughing gas party promised to provide fun. At the party, a shop assistant, Samuel Cooley, volunteered to inhale nitrous oxide. He became temporarily maniacal and chased another man around the room. As he did so, Cooley tripped and severely injured his leg. Wells interviewed the man later and was amazed to hear that Cooley did not feel his injury.

Wells went on to experiment on himself, asking a colleague to give him nitrous oxide before his colleague extracted one of Wells' own decayed teeth. Wells felt no pain at all. Horace Wells rushed to perform a demonstration at Harvard. His partner, William Thomas Green Morton (WTG Morton), assisted Wells in administering the nitrous oxide to a student needing a tooth extracted.

DOI: 10.1201/9781003324058-11

For whatever reason, insufficient nitrous oxide was given, and the extraction was not painless. The students hissed and the doctors booed. The hostile reception caused Wells to pack up and head the next day to Hartford, Connecticut. Later, Wells tested dental anesthesia again, using a much larger dose of nitrous oxide on a woman, but the patient almost died after a coma of several hours. This was the end for Wells, who voluntarily abandoned dentistry.[2]

On the other hand, WTG Morton, a tall, mustached, 25-year-old dentist when he assisted Wells, continued to pursue anesthesia. Morton stayed in Boston and achieved a reputation for crowning teeth with gold, a wonderful tooth-hardening procedure done by only a few dentists in 1845. Crowning a tooth was limited by the associated pain. Morton continued to struggle with the idea of painless dentistry and decided to audit courses at Harvard Medical School, hoping a knowledge of general therapeutics would help. Morton lodged with one of the professors there, Dr. Charles Jackson.

In the course of their association, Jackson told Morton about the pain-relieving properties of ether, and Morton used it locally on a tooth to relieve pain. Morton also became aware that when tuberculosis patients inhaled ether in small amounts, it eased their torment. Jackson did not wish to experiment with ether.

Recalling his nitrous oxide fiasco with Wells, Morton decided to experiment with ether before trying it on patients. He administered it to insects, fish, animals, and even his wife's pet dog. Finally, taking it himself and placing the ether on a handkerchief on September 30, 1846, he remained unconscious for eight minutes. He then gave the ether in the same way to one of his dental patients and extracted a tooth painlessly.[3]

Morton foresaw profit in his method and hurried to the Boston Patent Office. When Dr. Jackson heard of Morton's patent application, he demanded 10% of Morton's fees since he was the first to tell Morton of the properties of ether. Patients flooded Morton for painless extractions and gold crowning. His practice was so well attended that he could pay Jackson his 10% without undue hardship.

Morton left his dental work to his associates and turned his attention to the problem of extending anesthesia long enough for a surgical operation. Inhaling ether from a handkerchief was dangerous, as the amount inhaled could not be controlled. So, he devised an inhaler to overcome this difficulty (Figure 11.1). It was a glass globe filled with ether, fitted with two necks. The patient inhaled ether vapor by breathing in the long arm, and the tap in the short arm regulated the amount of air flowing into the globe. Thus, the amount of ether was precise and the depth and duration of anesthesia controlled.

After satisfying himself that the ether apparatus was safe and effective, Morton had trouble persuading any surgeon to permit its use. He encountered considerable opposition, no doubt much of it due to the fact that he was not a physician. Jackson, being a doctor, could have helped, but seemed only interested in collecting his 10% of Morton's fees.

Morton refused to give up and doggedly persisted. He eventually interested Dr. John Collins Warren, the senior surgeon, and one of the founders of Massachusetts General Hospital, where the elder surgeon had operated for 30 years.

Perhaps timing was the key. It is said Morton approached Warren just after the surgeon was unnerved by the cries of a young man whose leg he had amputated. Warren consented and scheduled an operation to remove a tumor from the neck of Gilbert Abbot, a 25-year-old thin man to which Morton could administer his ether.

The day arrived. October 16, 1846. The surgical pit at Massachusetts General Hospital had four semicircle observation rows rising above the floor of the

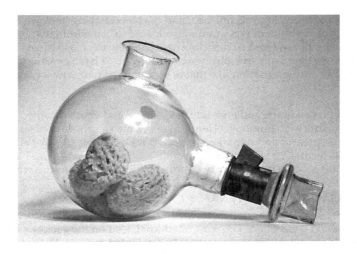

Figure 11.1 A replica of Morton's ether inhalation apparatus device. The right end attached to a face mask. The top opening was for insertion of the liquid ether. The sponges inside the globe helped to slowly release the ether. (From Wellcome.)

operating room, filled with the elite of Boston's surgeons. It had been announced that "a test of some preparation was to be made for which the astonishing claim had been made that it would render the person operated upon free from pain."

Gilbert Abbot was led into the operating room and strapped to the chair. An eyewitness described the early scene:

> Those present were incredulous, and, as Dr. Morton had not arrived at the time appointed and fifteen minutes had passed, Dr. Warren said, with significant meaning, "I presume he is otherwise engaged." This was followed with a "derisive laugh," and Dr. Warren grasped his knife and was about to proceed with the operation. At that moment, Dr. Morton entered a side door, when Dr. Warren turned to him and in a strong voice said, "Well, sir, your patient is ready."[4]

With an apology for detaining Dr. Warren and a statement that he had been compelled to wait for the completion of the newest version of his apparatus, Dr. Morton stepped to the bedside and asked Mr. Abbott, "Are you afraid?"

"No!" replied Abbot; "I feel confident and will do precisely as you tell me."

Raising the tube to his mouth, Abbot was sound asleep in four minutes. Dr. Morton then replied to Dr. Warren, "Your patient is ready, sir."[4]

Dr. Nathan Rice, the authorized biographer of WTG Morton, described the scene as follows:

> As Dr. Warren, seizing the bunch of veins in his hand, made the first incision through the skin, the patient made no sound nor moved one muscle of his body; as the operation progressed, all eyes were riveted on this novel scene in eager expectancy and amazement. The silence of the tomb reigned in the large amphitheater, and the form of each beholder was as still and immovable as the skeletons and mummies which hung in the cases behind them.

At length the operation was finished, and the blood having been washed from his face, the patient was gradually allowed to come from his anesthetic state. When fully restored to consciousness and able to answer questions, he gave the triumphant and gratifying intelligence, "I have experienced no pain, but only a sensation like that of scraping the part with a blunt instrument."[5]

Dr. Warren turned to the audience and said slowly and emphatically, "Gentleman, this is no humbug." Henry Bigelow, also a professor of surgery at Harvard, was present and remarked in part, "Our craft has, once for all, been robbed of its terrors."[4]

Warren and Morton performed two more painless operations the next day.

TROUBLES WITH THE PATENT

Difficulty arose as the Massachusetts Medical Society objected to Morton's patent on his secret concoction. This was unethical based on the society's rule that no physician should promote a secret and/or patented remedy. Morton acquiesced and revealed his substance as ether, thereby greatly reducing any profit to be made by himself.

News soon spread across the Atlantic to England, where Robert Liston performed the first major operation under ether in England on December 21, 1846. Liston had received news about ether through a friend's letter from Dr. Bigelow of Boston, who enthusiastically described Morton's success. Before the operation, the British surgeon was recorded saying dryly to the audience, "We are going to try a Yankee dodge today, gentlemen, for making men insensible."

After the leg amputation was performed, the patient awoke and asked, "When are you going to begin?" Liston exclaimed to the audience, "This Yankee dodge beats mesmerism hollow."[6]

Back in America, Morton eventually faced financial problems without a patent. In 1847, physicians from the Massachusetts General Hospital petitioned Congress for a financial award to be given to Morton. Despite the sponsorship of Daniel Webster and Oliver Wendell Holmes, the bill never passed (partly because of competing claims of discovery by others).

Jealous of the instant worldwide fame achieved by Morton, controversy soon erupted over the true discoverer of the use of ether for surgical anesthesia. Horace Wells claimed, by virtue of his failed demonstration earlier at Harvard, to be the first. Most have dismissed his claim because he did not persevere to convince others.

Charles Jackson later claimed Morton was his assistant. When asked why he, Jackson, was not present on the momentous day of October 16, 1846, Jackson disingenuously reported he was in Europe on more pressing business and had instructed his assistant, Dr. Morton, on what to do. Jackson is on record as having made other unrelated false claims, including inventing the telegraph machine (a claim later completely rejected by the US Supreme Court).

Crawford Long, a physician in Georgia, appears to have evidence of using ether as general anesthesia in 1842, four years before Morton. He used it for four operations and then inexplicably stopped using it. It is said superstitious villagers demanded Long cease and desist. In any case, Long did not publish his claims until 1849 and did not convince others to use it.

Morton went on to deliver ether anesthesia to more than 2,000 wounded federal soldiers at Fredericksburg and other battle locations during the Civil War. Morton's son posthumously published in 1904 a 15-page memoir written by his father about his voluntary Civil War experience using ether anesthesia. His Civil War writing is recommended for a viewpoint of the federal army and the beginnings of the modern battlefield hospital.[78]

Despite his beneficence to humanity in general and soldiers in particular, Morton was penniless and only 49 years old when he died of a stroke in 1868.

Ether was discovered in the sixteenth century. Why then did it take so long to realize its potential? This is not understood. Yet ether is an example of a therapy clearly beneficial. A controlled trial is not necessary since, certainly, no one would sign up for the control group. Statistics were not needed.

Few people realize today that general anesthesia allowed exploration of the abdomen and chest. Prior to 1846, invasion into these sterile cavities was painfully impossible. Coupled with advances in antisepsis for the operating room, a new age was to dawn with enormous advances in surgical treatment.

Sir William Osler, a leading American physician who examined the controversy over the discovery of ether in 1846, pointed out in 1913, "In science, the credit goes to the man who convinces the world, not the man to whom the idea first occurs." By this criterion, it was Morton who convinced the world that ether anesthesia for surgery would work.

NOTES

1 Rosen G. Mesmerism and surgery: A strange chapter in the history of anesthesia. *Journal of the History of Medicine and Allied Sciences* 1946;1; pp. 527–50.

2 Prescott F. *The Control of Pain.* London: English Universities Press; 1964, pp. 23–4.

3 Ibid, p. 25.

4 Society MM, Society NES. *Boston Medical and Surgical J* 1896;135; pp. 393–9.

5 Rice N. *Trials of a Public Benefactor* (reprint). Carlisle, MA: Applewood Books; 2010, p. 93.

6 Cock W. The first major operation under ether in England. *American Journal of Surgery: Quarterly Supplement of Anesthesia and Analgesia* 1915;29; pp. 98–101.

7 Morton WTG. *The Use of Ether as an Anesthetic at the Battle of the Wilderness in the Civil War.* Chicago: Press of American Medical Association; 1904.

8 Sturges, P. (director). *The Great Moment.* Movie. 1944. 83 minutes. (A dramatization of Morton's discovery, true to facts, with enjoyable acting by Joel McCrea.)

12 Tuberculosis, Streptomycin, and Robert Koch

"It is my death warrant!" exclaimed the physician-turned-poet John Keats, after coughing up blood in 1818. He well knew the "white death," so named for the pallor of severe anemia caused by frequent fits of pulmonary hemorrhage. It was also "white" from its long association with childhood, innocence, and even holiness. During the course of human history, conservative estimates suggest more than a billion people have died from this infection.[1] But we must not speak in the past tense since tuberculosis is alive and well, surviving the near knock-out punch antibiotics gave it in the 1950s. Tuberculosis persists as one of the most dangerous infectious diseases in the world today. More than a third of the world's population remains infected and often asymptomatic.

Skeletons from Neolithic burial grounds and Egyptian mummies show evidence of tuberculosis. The disease became so common in the 1600s that John Bunyan labeled it "the Captain of all these men of death." While death was not immediate, like the black plague, it nonetheless killed on a huge scale. Tuberculosis was ever present and lurking. Victims usually suffered a lingering death in about two to ten years.

The roll call of victims leads to the question of whether the knowledge of a shortened life led to intensive creativity: names such as Robert Louis Stevenson, Edgar Allen Poe, Chopin, Jane Austen, George Orwell, to cite a few.[2]

The cause was hotly debated until late in the nineteenth century. Before Koch's (discussed in this chapter) discovery of the responsible bacterium, virtually all northern European and US physicians felt the disease was a hereditary diathesis. A diathesis is a constitutional predisposition toward a diseased state. Dr. James Copland, a British physician, hypothesized in 1869 many precipitating causes of tuberculosis in those with the presumed diathesis. These unproven rules became enshrined in medical schools over the next 50 years. Most items represented deviations from "healthy living," such as "ill-regulated studies and an incontinent search for pleasure." Improper clothing of areas of the body that lowered body heat was another culprit—"immodest dress in women in particular could fatally expose their respiratory system."[3] Before the reader laughs, all mothers have told us to "wear your cap or you will catch cold."

Florence Nightingale had no doubts—she rarely had any on matters of health—and her words about bad air carried enormous weight. She believed that air rebreathed by too many people for too long could generate tuberculosis. Her convictions seemed vindicated when the incidence of disease in the army fell after the barracks were enlarged and new rules for ventilation enforced.[3]

But not all of Europe agreed with the diatheses or miasma theory. Since the 1700s, Italians considered tuberculosis a contagious disease. The belongings of any tubercular lodger in an apartment were burned after their departure. For example, the famous violinist Niccolo Paganini suffered a relapse of his tuberculosis during a concert tour in 1818 while living in Naples. As soon as the landlord deduced the nature of the illness, he turned the celebrated violinist into the street, hurling all his possessions after him. Paganini was fortunate that one of his admirers happened to be passing by and took him to more hospitable lodgings outside the city. However, the helper of Paganini had to convince the second frightened landlord by first beating him with a stick.[4]

The Ancient Greeks coined the term "phthisis" (literally, "wasting") for this disease. This label persisted until the early nineteenth century. In 1839, J. L. Schonlein, Professor of Medicine in Zurich, suggested the medical term "tuberculosis" as a generic name for all manifestations of phthisis since the tubercle (meaning a "nodule") appeared to be the fundamental pathological

DOI: 10.1201/9781003324058-12

unit. Since the fourteenth century, the most common lay term for phthisis in English has been "consumption."

Otherwise, the diagnosis of consumption was challenging to make, particularly in its initial stages, prior to the discovery of the bacterium.

Physicians divided tuberculosis into three stages. The earliest signs were so vague that it was impossible to determine with certainty that any particular person had consumption. A dry, persistent cough marks the first stage with mild breathing difficulties, particularly during exercise. Given the dire prognosis of tuberculosis, many physicians, and of course patients, were eager to avoid the label of "consumption" for as long as possible.

The second stage brings intense and debilitating symptoms. The cough becomes increasingly severe, frequent, and harassing. A fever spikes twice daily, along with a rapid pulse. The fever lends ruddiness to the complexion of consumptives, giving them a deceptive appearance of good health. During the second stage, ulcers appear in the throat, causing hoarseness and inability to eat or speak above a whisper.

Diagnosis becomes more certain in the third stage, where the lungs sound hollow. The cough, known as the "graveyard cough" or "death rattle," is distinctive and unmistakable. The three principle lung lesions (Figure 12.1) that could develop were an abscess (pocket of pus), consolidation (fluid filling the air spaces), and pulmonary artery irritation or arteritis (inflammation or irritation).

Outside the lungs, the fearsome problems of chronic fever and diarrhea lead to massive weight loss. The final appearance is ghostly and cadaveric, one epitomized by the term "consumption."

Fortunately, at least in view of the poignancy of deathbed conversations, the mental faculties maintain their integrity to the last. This allows the patient to say goodbye to their family and speak, however weakly, to the end. Pulmonary artery hemorrhage, manifested by coughing up blood, is often the terminal event.

ROBERT KOCH

The first momentous discovery in tuberculosis took place in Berlin, Germany. On the evening of March 24, 1882, a small man with spectacles named Robert Koch (pronounced "coke") announced his findings. Robert Koch (1843–1910) was born in Clausthal in the Harz Mountains, the most northern mountain range in Germany. Koch graduated with honors at the University of Gottingen, a leading medical school at the time. As a resident physician in Hamburg, he met Emmy Fraatz, who agreed to marry him on the condition that he abandon his secret ambitions—exploring the South Sea Islands and winning the Iron Cross in battle. Instead, he should pursue a more humdrum prospect of a rural general practice.

Koch performed his medical rounds on horseback for several years in the small Prussian town of Wollstein. He attended farmers, farmer's wives, their babies, and often their dogs and cats. Apart from reading the leading German medical journals once a week, he was completely cut off from developments in medicine or science. But on his 28th birthday, Frau Emmy surprised him with a present to change their lives. She gave him a microscope of modest capacity. The type bought today for bright 10 year olds to awaken their minds to the wonders of the natural world.

In the spare time snatched from a busy general practice, Koch taught himself the rudiments of microbiological research. Koch's first microbiological interest was one that had also excited Louis Pasteur—anthrax. Anthrax is a savage

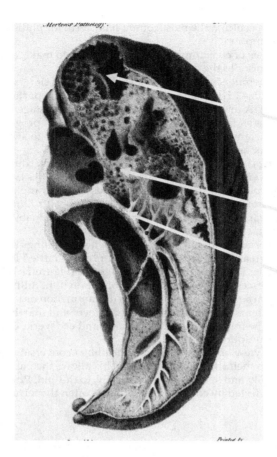

Figure 12.1 A drawing from 1834 of a coronal section of advanced pulmonary tuberculosis. The top line indicates an apical cavitation. This is very typical of advanced pulmonary tuberculosis. The middle line points to a pneumonia process where white blood cells are attacking the TB bacteria and filling up the air space with fluid and debris rather than functional air. The lower line points to an arteritis or an inflamed pulmonary artery. It is these blood vessels that can rupture and lead to voluminous bleeding, as evidenced by coughing up blood. This is often a fatal complication. (From Wellcome Library, London. Attribution, Public Domain Mark.)

disease, and it was then a poorly understood killer of sheep and sometimes man. It had many characteristics, suggesting microbial transmission.

Koch made every tool he needed. He built his own cages and took care of his menagerie of experimental animals. Koch often had to improvise techniques. Some of his early creations, like the hanging drop preparation, are still in use. In many respects, the antithesis of Pasteur, Koch was meticulous to a fault, wary of jumping to conclusions, and critical of his own results. He determinedly avoided shortcuts that might lead him astray.

It took Koch six years in the wilderness before he was satisfied with his findings on anthrax. He emerged from isolation and took his notes and microscopic slides to the University of Breslau (now Wroclaw). Here Koch achieved instant academic success. Professors at the university recognized the importance of his work on anthrax and helped obtain a research position for him. Seven years earlier, Louis Pasteur had flamboyantly predicted that science would soon be ready to eliminate all microbial diseases. Koch's work on anthrax added a new element of reality to this prospect. Not only did he establish that the disease was caused by a single, identifiable bacillus. He also demonstrated how anthrax spores could remain dormant under extreme adverse conditions—in dead and buried carcasses, for example, only to revive and start to multiply when transferred to new living hosts and kill again. The term "spore," meaning seed, was ancient, but Koch's demonstration of anthrax spores was the first time their nature and importance were established in modern microbiology.

Koch then turned his attention to tuberculosis. He began by injecting material obtained from a young man, who had recently died from acute tuberculosis, into guinea pigs and then into rabbits. Within a few months, he caught his first microscopic glimpse of small, slender, and fragile rods he suspected as the cause of tuberculosis. Koch, reluctant to prematurely report a discovery, continued to gather data for more than a year.

Koch did not pursue his research unimpeded. Rudolph Virchow, a famous pathologist and doctor who was regarded as the leading physician in Germany, opposed Koch's ideas. Medical research throughout Germany was so dominated by Virchow that his word was taken as gospel. Virchow had recently rejected Koch's (and Pasteur's) theories of the bacterial cause of disease. Nevertheless, Koch's work was rewarded in 1880 when he was appointed to a post at the Imperial Health Office in Berlin. The establishment of the Imperial Health Office to specifically attract Koch was regarded as a personal affront by Virchow, who shunned Koch.

KOCH PRESENTS HIS FINDINGS—MARCH 24, 1882

Because of Virchow's opposition, the momentous lecture of March 24, 1882, took place in a physiological institute, not the school of medicine.[5] The evening would also have another eventual Nobel Prize winner in attendance, Dr. Paul Ehrlich, who would discover the first modestly effective agent against syphilis, agent 606 (so named for his 606th experiment).

As Koch rose to speak, he fumbled nervously with his papers. Shortsighted, he had to peer closely into those same papers as he began to read. In the words of one observer, "Koch was by no means a dynamic lecturer who would overwhelm his audience with brilliant words. He spoke slowly and haltingly, but what he said was clear, simple, logically stated—in short, clear, unadulterated gold."[6]

Koch stated,

The nature of tuberculosis has been studied by many, but this has led to no successful results. Those staining methods which have been so useful in the demonstration of microorganisms in other diseases have been unsuccessful here. Every experiment devised for the isolation and culture of the infective agent of tuberculosis has also failed. In my own studies on tuberculosis, I began by using those same methods without success. Several causal observations have induced me to throw away these methods and to strike out in a new direction which has finally led to positive results. The proof is possible through a certain staining procedure which has allowed the discovery of characteristic, although previously undescribed, bacteria in organs which have been altered by tuberculosis.[6]

A rush of excited murmurings must have interrupted his presentation. Observers would later describe the increasing excitement with which the audience followed every step of his work. Koch well realized the enormity of what he had disclosed. Yet, those describing the speech later would remark on how Koch's face remained passive throughout. He had, he continued calmly, been forced to invent a new manner of staining.

Koch went on to describe the fact that he would stain tissue on his microscopic slides with a dye, methylene blue, developed by Paul Erlich. Everybody in the audience was familiar with methylene blue, but this particular stain caused all the tissue to turn deep blue. This made it difficult to pick out any fine detail, such as a tiny bacterium. Koch related he had overcome the problem by pouring over his glass slides a counterstain. Yet, it was necessary, he explained, not only to add the second dye, Vesuvin, but also that the slide needed to be heated for several minutes. Now, under the microscope, the structures of the animal tissues would appear brown, while the tubercule bacteria would be a beautiful blue. Indeed, all the other bacteria, except the tubercle bacillus, would assume a brown color. He went on to say that with "the color contrast between the brown colored tissues and the blue bacteria, the bacteria, although present in small numbers, are easy to find and recognize."[7]

Modern staining for tuberculosis uses different stains. Nonetheless, the use of a counterstain to visualize tuberculosis bacteria was Koch's key discovery. The audience gazed at Koch in unconcealed amazement, every one of them was a doctor or scientist for whom the cause of tuberculosis was the greatest mystery. Koch had brought his entire laboratory to the lecture hall that night: his microscopes, test tubes with cultures, and his microscopic slides of animal tissue preserved in alcohol. Koch asked them to check his findings for themselves. He expected them to do so—as indeed these trained scientists would.

Koch went on that evening to relate three famous postulates, which have been memorized by every medical student since. These postulates, in his opinion, had to be fulfilled before a cause-and-effect relationship between a germ and disease could be proven. These postulates were: one, the organism must be found in every pathological lesion; two, this organism should be capable of being cultivated pure outside the body for several generations; three, after a pure culture for a sufficient length of time was maintained for several generations, it should be able to reproduce the original illness in laboratory animals.

Koch concluded,

All these facts taken together can lead to only one conclusion: that the bacilli which are present in tuberculosis substances not only accompany the tuberculosis process but are the cause of it. In the bacilli, we have the actual infective cause of tuberculosis.[5]

Reaction at the end of this speech was strange and baffling to Koch. Where one would have expected applause or at least some heated questioning, there was a stunned silence.

Paul Erlich would later confess he could barely contain his own excitement: "I hold that evening to be the most important experience of my life."[5]

The news traveled quickly considering the era. Koch's written paper was published in a Berlin clinical journal on April 10, and on the same day, a copy of it landed on the desk of the eminent British scientist, John Tyndale, in London. Realizing its importance, he summarized its main findings in a letter to the *Times*, which published it on April 22, 1882. The next day, the *New York World* carried a brief cable dispatch announcing the discovery, and two days later, both the *New York Times* and the *New York Tribune* published Tyndale's letter in full.[5]

Skepticism reigned for a few months. Soon, European scientists began reproducing Koch's discovery, and his concepts were soon accepted. But there was still no proven treatment.

TREATMENT QUACKERY

One of the earliest disease manifestations described was "the King's Evil." This term refers to golf-ball-sized lymph nodes in the neck due to tuberculosis. This condition could lead to terrible ulceration and scarring. Called the King's Evil, it was also known as "scrofula" (meaning "little pigs"). Medieval commentators recognized it as a manifestation of a general disease with poor prognosis. Why it was considered susceptible to the touch of kings is uncertain, but it was so identified as early as the fifth century. The touch was the basis of treatment and, indeed, if contemporary chronicles are to be believed, of numerous cures in most of Europe. However, it is odd that royalty themselves were not immune. That both England's Edward VI and France's Charles IX were scrofulous and may have died from tuberculosis in no way diminished the conviction of their subjects.

Records provide a guide to the prevalence of the condition. Edward I (1272–1307) touched 533 sufferers in one month. This practice continued even until the 1700s. Charles II during his 25-year reign (1660–1685) is said to have touched 92,102 of his subjects. It is difficult to understand how the King's touch healed.[8]

Layfolk also had their surefire cures. In Britain, they believed in the inhalation of the exhaled warm breath of healthy animals. In Suffolk, the source had to be a stallion. In the Scottish Lowlands, it was a cow. And in the highlands, the breath of a sheep.[10]

DOCTORS DECEIVED

In contrast to the scientific approach to diagnosis in the nineteenth century, the treatment quackery of tuberculosis was rooted in the flimsiest evidence. These ineffective treatments were especially believed when expounded by medical practitioners. One physician, having observed what he thought was the immunity of butchers to consumption, claimed total success with four advanced cases of tuberculosis by rubbing lard into their bodies. Another variant was chaulmoogra oil (foul-tasting, foul-smelling liquid imported from Burma) applied both externally and given by mouth. Many patients presumably felt that so obnoxious of a treatment had to be effective.[9]

Doctors both in Britain and Europe sought to get at the disease with inhalations. Dr. Reid Clanny in Britain pumped 12 cubic inches of sulfur, hydrogen, and coal gas into a woman's lungs four times a day for six weeks. Supposedly, after a fortnight, all her symptoms disappeared. (A rival practitioner informed readers of the medical journal *Lancet* that the patient never had tuberculosis in the first place). Fantastic ways to administer the gas were then developed. In German-speaking countries, the emphasis was more on the temperature of the gas than its composition. After it was shown in the 1880s that most pathogenic organisms could not survive high temperatures, pumping into the rectum of air superheated to 150°F became fashionable. Excellent results were claimed![10,11]

Even the cautious Robert Koch in 1900 announced at the Tenth International Congress of Medicine in Berlin that he had discovered a substance that could "in some cases" protect against tuberculosis and "under certain circumstances" cure the disease. The material, called Koch's Lymph, had proteins from killed bacteria harvested from infected guinea pigs. This was a breathtaking announcement. Consumptives traveled in droves to Berlin to get any chance of being treated with this wonder medicine. But further testing showed it was ineffective. Why the normally cautious Koch would declare such a preliminary finding prematurely has never been explained. For a time in the early 1900s, the reputation of Koch hung in the balance. Rumors circulated that he had accepted a bribe of a million marks from his government, which was anxious to bask in his reflected glory and trumpet Germany's preeminence in science around the world.

Nobody that knew him believed it, but upheavals in his private life gave the calumny a veneer of credibility. He had fallen in love with a pretty and gifted art student, Hedwig Freiberg (32 years his junior), and the liaison could not be kept secret. He obtained a divorce from Emmy, his wife of 28 years, and set out on an around-the-world honeymoon with his new bride. Despite his reputation as a talented scientist, scandal could have ruined him, but the imperial government ruthlessly suppressed it.

On his return, the Kaiser decorated him with the order of the Crown and Star. He then became the director of the Institute of Infectious Diseases (now named after him) and traveled to Africa and India, making valuable contributions to the cause of cholera, typhoid, and sleeping sickness. In 1905, he received the Nobel Prize for his work in tuberculosis.[12]

Other physicians made similar mistakes based on minimal evidence. In the 1920s, calcium treatment enjoyed a thread of evidence. The observation that healed tubercular lesions often underwent calcification on chest radiographs led a French physician Louis Renon, in 1906, to report that in a village with many lime-burning furnaces, there had been no cases of tuberculosis. He suggested the inhalation of small calcium-lime particles was the reason for the lack of tuberculosis. Several other physicians in the United States and abroad also investigated similar areas, and soon recommended calcium in any form might be helpful. Later, better-designed studies found no evidence to support such an assertion.[13]

Calcium was at least cheap and, in moderation, lacked any deleterious effects. Neither could be said about one of the most trumpeted, but useless, chemicals advocated in the 1920s—gold. While gold had been used for hundreds of years in different human ailments, its place in treatment owed more to glitter than to experimental evidence. In 1890, Koch gave it a slight breath of scientific respect when in a preliminary report he wrote that gold cyanides slightly inhibited the growth of tubercle bacilli in cultures. Several animal studies followed up on the finding, which concluded that gold appeared to promote rather than inhibit tuberculosis in living animals.[13]

Despite this animal evidence, several physicians around the world began promoting gold salts. The most notable one was Dr. Mollgäard at the University of Copenhagen. He had discovered a complex gold salt, which he claimed had a specific beneficial action in tuberculosis. He christened the patented compound Sanocrysin. When other scientists studied this, it seemed like the animals usually died from shock or high fevers. Dr. Mollgäard attributed these side effects to toxins released after the tubercle bacilli were killed.

Two actions caused the downfall of Sanocrysin. A controlled American trial, reported in 1931, showed no effect of Sanocrysin on tuberculosis. Moreover, 1 of 12 treated patients died from liver failure and all had kidney damage, while all 12 control subjects had no kidney or liver toxicity (Chapter 17). This expensive therapy eventually faded away after 1935, when it was reported that Mollgäard had fudged his results by failing to report that his first batch of experimental guinea pigs had been infected with a weakened strain of tuberculosis.[13]

One effective drug, at least for comfort, which physicians used since the sixteenth century, was laudanum. This was an opiate drug that by the early 1800s was more purified in the form of morphine. It was a mild sedative and analgesic that allowed sufferers to tolerate intense pain. As a result, millions of tuberculosis patients died peacefully in the arms of their loved ones.

In the context of tuberculosis, few worried about the risk of addiction. Laudanum and other opiates have one potent side effect—namely, severe constipation. However, doctors have always excelled in purgation, and laudanum gave them a chance to show their virtuosity.

SOCIAL OUTLOOK FOR PATIENTS

During most of the nineteenth century, men and women with chronic tuberculosis were labeled invalids. The term originated in the seventeenth century to identify soldiers and sailors unfit for active duty. Because of their wounds or loss of limb, invalids were excused from military service and often given a pension. But by the nineteenth century, the term encompassed all persons, military or civilian, that were weakened by disease and lacked the strength to participate fully in daily activities. Invalidism was as much a social as a medical category. To be classified as invalid was to be excused from fully complying with social expectations. Invalids were allowed to modify, or in the extreme case, to avoid the obligation to earn an income or fulfill the duties of wife and mother. Yet, invalids had a primary duty to meet—they had the "life-long occupation of improving."[14]

Invalids had difficulty planning their lives. Some people with tuberculosis died quickly (within months), but many suffered a severe attack followed by respite lasting 10, 20, or even 30 years. How could one plan a career or think about marriage and children? The dilemma was frustrating. Was it necessary to change their perspective career? More poignantly, should invalids avoid engagement and marriage?

Religion and social mores provided some answers, particularly as they distinguished between duties (that is marriage and childbearing) and privileges (higher education and a professional calling). Because marriage was a duty, the answer to the question of whether to avoid it was a resounding no. Thus, when the aunt of Jane Pierce (the president's wife) was engaged to be married to a consumptive widower with three grown children, a friend wrote that if the groom's health should be restored, he would be an excellent husband (but such a fate seemed "extremely doubtful"). In fact, he died soon after the wedding. Similarly, no one made adverse judgments when Ralph Waldo Emerson married Ellen Tucker when she was in the final stage of consumption. Indeed, it was commonplace in popular literature for a bride to die of consumption on or immediately after the wedding day, with the bridal dress turned into a shroud or a winding sheet.[14]

GO WEST AND BREATHE AGAIN

Tuberculosis was a key theme in the settlement of the American west. Beginning in the 1840s and then gathering momentum in the latter part of the century, men and women with symptoms of consumption moved to the mountains and deserts of the west. By 1900, one-quarter of the migration to California and one-third to Colorado sought to overcome tuberculosis. One railway company's slogan was, "Go west and breathe again." An editor of a Southern California newspaper wrote, "Men go west not to buy land, but to buy lungs."[15]

While most states west of the Mississippi had communities founded and developed for health seekers, Colorado and Southern California in particular were significant in this regard. More than half of the residents of Pasadena, California, Colorado Springs and Denver, Colorado, came directly as a result of tuberculosis, either in themselves or in their parents or grandparents.[15]

As more invalids traveled west, narratives about their experiences proliferated. Their advocacy that health would return was clear. In fact, so much so that in Mark Twain's *Roughing It*, the topic was prime for satire. "The air up here (Lake Tahoe) in the clouds is very pure and fine, bracing and delicious. And why shouldn't it be? It is the same air the angels breathe."[16]

He went on to relate,

I know a man who went there to die, but he made a failure of it. He was a skeleton when he came and could barely stand…three months later he was sleeping out-of-doors regularly, eating all he could hold three times a day, and chasing game over mountains 3,000 feet high for recreation. And he was a skeleton no longer but weighed part of a ton. This is no fancy sketch but the truth. His disease was consumption. I fully recommend his experience to other skeletons.[16]

Health seekers to the west appreciated there was no stigma to their disease. The fit even sympathized with them. The *Colorado Springs Gazette* stated in 1873, "They (consumptives) are drowning men clutching at straws and are worthy of our sincerest sympathy."

The town of Pasadena, California, was founded solely for tuberculosis patients. In 1873, a frail D. M. Berry arrived as a scout for a group of consumptives from Indiana. Berry, who suffered from severe respiratory ailments, had not slept well for years. At night, he had so much difficulty that he would awake and remain sitting in a chair until the next morning. On his first night in Pasadena, he slept soundly and awoke the next morning refreshed. He was known to repeat the story and exclaim, "Do you know, sir, that last night is the first night in three years that I have remained in bed all night?" Berry found the site he was looking for. The Indiana Colony, as Pasadena was first called, was composed of Midwesterners that went to sunny California to benefit the health of someone in their family. By 1886, the colony had grown into a small city.[15]

Pasadena did not cure everyone. Those with advanced stages rambled the streets aimless and helpless. Walking to the post office in Pasadena was unnerving. As one observer said, "These poor wanderers, driven from home by failing health, congregate about the doors, sit coughing about the steps or lean upon the walls with eager anxious faces, waiting, hoping for letters from home."[17]

Since there has not been a controlled trial of tuberculosis patients in the dry, sunny west versus the eastern United States, we will never know if these patients were helped by moving west. However, the tuberculosis bacillus requires a high-oxygen environment, and this is the reason it is so often in the lungs. Perhaps the high altitude and lower oxygen content of Colorado air effectively reduced multiplication of the bacteria. The alternative to moving west was to enter a sanitarium. The sanitarium movement mushroomed from the mid-nineteenth century until World War II when effective chemotherapy became available. In 1900, the United States had 34 sanitariums with 4,400 beds. In 1925, numbers had risen to 536 sanitariums with 73,000 beds.

In the sanitarium, the invalid became a patient again. Strict bed rest (i.e., bedpan use) was the first order of the admission. An attendant spoon-fed meals. Even though confined, the bed could be wheeled out to the sunshine. After two to six months, the patient began to exercise and stroll outdoors. Belief that pure air was helpful continued to be part of the sanitarium treatment, even after the tuberculosis bacillus was discovered. Old theories die slowly.

It is difficult to know if the sanitarium movement produced any benefit. No controlled trials of sanitarium placement versus home exist. Superficially, the results appeared better than staying home. But, by definition, sanitariums took only "early" cases; these cases were more likely to recover with or without treatment. One obvious benefit of patients staying in a sanitarium for years is that they were separated from the community (i.e., quarantined) and thus unable to transmit infection. Indeed, there was a gradual but steady reduction of tuberculosis in Europe and the United States from the mid-nineteenth century until World War II. One exception was the spike in cases around World War I because of the chaos of social dislocation and crowding.

STREPTOMYCIN

Selman Waksman discovered the first effective antibiotic against tuberculosis. Selman was born on July 8, 1888, six years after the famous lecture by Koch in Berlin. He started life in a small farming community in Ukraine. After the death of his parents, Selman, at age 22, immigrated to the United States to live on a farm in New Jersey. He then enrolled at the nearby agricultural college named Rutgers, where he graduated with a bachelor of science degree in 1915. He continued his education and returned to Rutgers with a doctorate in soil microbiology.

For years, Dr. Waksman had observed that there was something in soil that killed the tubercle bacillus. It was difficult to determine the exact organism responsible. A graduate student named Albert Schatz joined Dr. Waksman and took on as his doctoral thesis the discovery of this inhibiting organism. Schatz centered on a group of anti-tuberculosis bacteria named *Actinomyces*. For months, the graduate student streaked growth plates of *Actinomyces* in one direction and placed colonies of non-tuberculosis bacteria at right angles. Discovering one strain that appeared effective in general against bacteria, they tested it against the slow-growing tuberculosis. After months of exhausting labor and 18-hour days, Schatz and Waksman found a strain that inhibited the tubercle bacillus. Waksman renamed this strain Streptomyces. From this organism, they derived a substance named streptomycin.

Waksman and his group anxiously awaited the trials of streptomycin in animals since so many possible antibiotics (a term coined by Waksman from Pasteur's idea of "antibiosis") had proven toxic in animals. However, this time, in animals, and subsequently in human subjects at the Mayo Clinic, streptomycin produced profound inhibition of the tuberculosis bacillus without apparent toxicity.

Waksman had a challenging time convincing George Merck in 1944 to produce testable quantities of streptomycin. The Merck Company was deeply committed to wartime production of penicillin. But intervention by Feldman and Hinshaw from the Mayo Clinic, who said more people died in the World War I from tuberculosis than in battle, along with the demonstrations of test tube efficacy, finally caused George Merck to commit resources that eventually would involve 50 scientists. "Had Merck not consented to do this at this time, the clinical evaluations of streptomycin would have been long delayed."[18] The obvious initial effectiveness also prompted Merck to give an amount of streptomycin valued at a million dollars (in 1940 value) to the American Research Council so they could start the monumental trial involving thousands of patients and hundreds of investigators.[19]

The testing of streptomycin for the treatment of tuberculosis formed one of the first randomized, controlled trials. In the first trial, it was noted that 27% of control (untreated) patients died, while only 7% of those on streptomycin did (Chapter 18). Within two years of its discovery, streptomycin proved to be a breakthrough in the treatment of tuberculosis. Patients with extensive disease responded dramatically by clearing their chest X-ray completely. Labeled as cured, they soon went home. But not every patient with tuberculosis was cured by it. Predictably, the long-standing, fibrotic lung disease proved the most resistant. In 1951, Selman Waksman received the Nobel Prize for his effort in discovering the first effective antibiotic in the treatment of tuberculosis.

After several years, in a frightening revelation of the future, doctors began to notice relapsed cases that did not respond to streptomycin a second time. The specter of drug resistance was emerging. Even today, this continues to be the primary problem with the treatment of tuberculosis.

PARA-AMINOSALICYLIC ACID—PAS

At the same time as Waksman's work, and unknown to him, a different approach to the treatment of tuberculosis was undertaken. Dr. Jorgen Lehmann, in Sweden, developed a derivative of the simple aspirin molecule, known as PAS or para-aminosalicylic acid. What led to the idea of Dr. Lehman considering that this compound could be a potential anti-tuberculosis drug was the seminal observation of a single-page paper in *Nature* in 1940. Dr. Bernheim, the author, reported experiments that revealed that when aspirin was added to a culture of tuberculosis bacilli, the germs doubled their oxygen uptake.

While thousands of scientists worldwide failed to appreciate this simple observation, Dr. Lehmann seized the clue. Most believed the waxy coat of the tubercle bacillus would not allow any drug to penetrate its shell. The Swedish doctor thought this was absurd, as the organism had to take up molecules of food and oxygen to live. He realized aspirin was passing into the tuberculosis bacillus and stimulating its growth. Dr. Lehmann reasoned that if he could change the structure of the aspirin, he could trick the organism into accepting a dysfunctional substitute. Follow-up experiments showed the inhibitor PAS was indeed taken up by the tubercle bacillus and served to poison it.[20]

Similar success in treating animals and humans was to be forthcoming. PAS was not as strong as streptomycin. And, like streptomycin, resistance to the PAS would appear several years after the drug was introduced. Single-drug resistance led to the treatment in the early 1950s of using both drugs at once. This combination was far more effective than either drug alone. It also helped cut down drug resistance.

Combination therapy is needed because the tubercle bacillus is always mutating. Since there are approximately one million bacilli in any given patient, there would usually be over the course of a year, a single bacterial mutant that would be resistant to a particular drug. Yet that particular individual bacterium would still be susceptible to a second drug. If a second drug were not given, the mutant bacterium would grow and form the basis of a relapse of tuberculosis in an affected patient.

CONCLUSION

The development of antibiotics against tuberculosis in the late 1940s and early 1950s resulted in all sanitariums emptying their patients. Patients began to receive antibiotics in the outpatient setting. As of this writing, treatment may be needed for up to 18 months. Given the lengthy treatment, compliance is a challenge. Missing doses of antibiotics can lead to drug-resistant tuberculosis. The number of drugs that can be used is limited, with few new ones on the horizon.

The situation has improved dramatically for the United States. The number of TB cases in 1900 was 175,000 (total population 76 million). In 2020, 7,800 cases were diagnosed in the United States, two-thirds of which were imported (total population 330 million). The problem for the United States is importation.[21] The number of people diagnosed with tuberculosis worldwide in 2020 was 10 million.[22] Most deaths involving TB are occurring in Africa and Southeast Asia.[23]

In contrast to the situation in the United States, it is unrealistic to even contemplate the global elimination of tuberculosis with available interventions since more than a third of the world's population is infected with latent[24] or chronic infection. However, our active participation in global programs to control tuberculosis is a responsibility. It will also help us reduce the chance of importing the "[c]aptain of all these men of death."

NOTES

1 Ryan F. *The Forgotten Plague: How the Battle against Tuberculosis Was Won—and Lost*. Boston: Little, Brown; 1992, p. 3.

2 Moorman LJ. *Tuberculosis and Genius*. Chicago: University of Chicago Press; 1940.

3 Dormandy T. *The White Death: A History of Tuberculosis*. Stockton, England: Hambledon Press; 1999; pp. 42–4.

4 Ibid, pp. 52–3.

5 Brock TD. *Robert Koch: A Life in Medicine and Bacteriology*. Washington, DC: American Society of Microbiology; 1999, pp. 117–39.

6 Ryan, pp. 10–1.

7 Ryan, p. 12.

8 Dormandy, p. 4.

9 Rogers L. Chaulmoogra oil in tuberculosis. *British Medical Journal* 1922;2; p. 703.

10 Dormandy, pp. 47–8.

11 To pump gas into the rectum seems untenable since it does not directly enter the lungs. The background reasoning would be that the WHDW, or rotten stuff, originated here (Chapter 1).

12 Dormandy, p 144.

13 Dormandy, pp. 267–72.

14 Rothman S. *Living in the Shadow of Death: Tuberculosis and the Social Experience of Illness in American History*. New York: Harper-Collins; 1994, p. 24.

15 Ibid, pp. 131–47.

16 Twain M. *Roughing It*. Google: Harper & Brothers; 1913, p. 158.

17 Rothman, p. 166.

18 Ryan, p. 234.

19 Ryan, p. 282.

20 Ryan, pp. 242–4.

21 Filardo TD, Feng P, Pratt RH, Price SF, Self JL. Tuberculosis—United States, 2021. *MMWR Morb Mortal Wkly Rep* 2022;71; pp. 441–6. DOI: 10.15585/mmwr.mm7112a1externalicon

22 This number reflects only mono-infection with TB and excludes HIV coinfection; coinfection would swell the number to 30%–50% higher or more, but patients dying with HIV often do not have the TB component cited by authorities. This remains a staggering number. If we had a military war with these many deaths, it would be considered catastrophic. The news media are virtually silent on this issue.

23 *Global Tuberculosis Report 2021*. Geneva: World Health Organization; 2021. License: CC BY-NC-SA 3.0 IGO.

24 Latent tuberculosis occurs when a person is infected with Mycobacterium tuberculosis but does not have active disease. Patients with latent tuberculosis are not contagious. About 10% of these people (5% in the first two years after infection and 0.1% per year thereafter) will go on to develop active tuberculosis (i.e., become contagious and damage body organs). If detected, latent TB can be easily treated and the dormant infection eliminated.

13 Placebo or the I Feel Better Pill

PLACEBO: THE SOMETIMES WONDERFUL DRUG

"Wow! Doc, I don't know what pill you gave me, but it made me so woozy, that I staggered for 30 minutes after I took it. I never want to take that medicine again!"

The effect of the first placebo I gave startled me. A placebo is an inert substance or sugar pill known to be without therapeutic effect. (Placebo means "I will please" in Latin.) The patient was a middle-aged male with vague symptoms of lightheadedness. After a thorough workup, my neurology consultant could not identify any abnormality. The patient implored me almost daily to do something. Given the absence of significant disease, I imagined a placebo might be helpful. I expected nothing would happen. I was wrong.

PLACEBOS AND SURGERY

Two surgical trials inform us about the power of placebo. One trial investigated serious heart pain called angina pectoris. The second concerned knee arthritis.

Angina pectoris is serious chest pain specific to the heart and occurs due to low oxygen levels. Partial blockages in coronary arteries that supply the heart are the culprit. Anginal pain occurs with objective changes in the electrocardiogram, known as "S-T elevations."

Italian researchers reported their findings with internal mammary artery ligation in the 1950s. The procedure reduced pain in 91% of cases of angina. Patients also used fewer nitroglycerine tablets. Nitroglycerine is a medicine that helps dilate coronary arteries and relieve angina. For comparison, spontaneous remission of angina pectoris ranges from 14%–19%.[1] Hundreds of thousands of patients rushed for this novel surgery.

The theory behind this operation seemed dubious to many. The internal mammary arteries (IMA) do not supply the heart, but only the chest wall. The operation involves incisions into the chest muscle in the second intercostal (rib) space. Then, the surgeon ties the IMA off. Interruption of the IMA was presumed to divert more blood into the coronary arteries.[1] The operation appealed since it did not involve invasion of the chest cavity. Opening the chest was a hazardous undertaking in the 1950s. Best of all, recovery from the minor procedure was immediate. Coronary angiography (inserting a catheter into the artery and placing contrast to check flow rates) was unavailable at the time.

Dr. Dimond from the University of Missouri challenged this idea in 1960. A sham operation was compared to ligation of the IMA in patients with angina pectoris. He studied a sham group of 5 patients and compared them to 13 IMA-ligated patients. Research candidates needed S-T elevations on their electrocardiogram tracings during episodes of angina. The sham group underwent skin and muscle incisions. But the IMA were untouched. Neither the patients nor the cardiologists knew who received the ligation.[2] This is an example of a double-blind study. Pain relief was identical between the two arms. Either procedure did not alter the exercise electrocardiogram.

One study note from the research study is of interest. The interviewer recorded from a sham patient:

I had a brief episode of burning pain in my incision yesterday while walking. ... Otherwise, I have had no other pain. I feel much better." The office note for the sham patient on the following day read: "The patient dropped dead today following moderate exertion."[2]

DOI: 10.1201/9781003324058-13

A year later, L. A. Cobb's group (University of Washington, Seattle), reproduced the findings of the Kansas group. Their sham group performed as well as the ligated group.[3] Use of the ligation operation for angina faded away. In an interview, L.A. Cobb was asked, "If the patient got all that much better (with the operation], why not do it?" His answer, "If something does not have a scientific or physiological basis, we generally do not adopt it, particularly for a surgical procedure."[4]

Even though a patient feels better from a placebo, there is no change in the underlying disease. When the disease fails to improve, survival does not change. Sham patient number two discussed earlier illustrates this idea. The damaged ship is sinking, but the captain smiles because he feels good about the situation. Or the disease is getting worse, but the patient thinks they are improving because they feel better.

KNEE OSTEOARTHRITIS

Osteoarthritis of the knee is a widespread problem. It occurs in more than 6% of the US population over age 30. Osteoarthritis consists of thinning of the cartilage or cushion between the solid bone surfaces of a joint. There are often crystals of cartilage or calcium phosphate within the joint.

Medical treatments may not relieve severe cases. The surgical alternative, called a lavage, is to insert a needle into the knee joint. Infusion of liters of saline and its drainage follow. This became a popular treatment in the United States in the 1990s. The year 2001 saw 660,000 knee lavage operations performed. In theory, such a procedure has common sense and rational appeal. The removal of debris within the knee joint should decrease inflammation. This ought to lessen pain and dysfunction of the knee.

Dr. Moseley (Baylor College of Medicine), in 2005, reported a placebo-controlled trial of arthroscopic surgery for knee osteoarthritis.[5] Sham arm patients were taken into the operating room and given intravenous sedation (not general anesthesia). The knee was made ready, and three 1 cm incisions were made in the skin as for a real lavage. The surgeon manipulated the knee as if arthroscopy was being performed. Splashing sounds of the lavage saline were simulated. No instruments entered the joint space. The patient stayed in the operating room for the same time needed for a debridement. The study had a robust design, in that one surgeon performed all the procedures. He was also not involved in the postoperative evaluation.

The follow-up study personnel were unaware of the treatment and placebo group assignments. Data about functional knee status were collected for two years.

For any parameter, there was no difference between the group that received the 10-liter lavage and those that did not. Pain scores decreased by about 20% in both groups and were maintained for the two-year follow-up. Yet, objective function was worse in the debridement group than in the placebo group.[5] The results suggest that the effects of debris on symptoms in an osteoarthritic joint are negligible. As one commenter put it, "Debridement and lavage may simply remove some evidence while the destructive forces of osteoarthritis continue to work."[6]

Furthermore, the implications of Moseley's work are much more than debunking a treatment. It serves to free up the field of research on osteoarthritis caught up with irrelevant debris. Flotsam that obscured our understanding of the more important causes of this disabling disease.

Controlled trials of surgery for angina and knee osteoarthritis provide valuable corrective knowledge. Yet, few sham surgical trials are reported.

Surgery has a powerful placebo effect. Consider how impressive the preoperative ritual is:

> The patient steps into a large hospital. The surgical team projects confidence. A consent is signed. The patient enters the operating cathedral, where green angels of care tend to basic needs. The anesthetist prepares the patient for temporary oblivion. The preoperative medication is given. These rituals are ideal for a placebo effect.[7]

THE PLACEBO EFFECT

Like many others, this author has been uneasy in using placebos. Charging a patient for an inert pill seems misspent money. Or is there a degree of dishonesty in giving a pill known not to work so a patient can feel better?

What about this phenomenon that can give complete relief of pain in 20%–80% of patients? Or why does an inert pill cause one out of every ten patients to have nausea? Or 1 patient in 20 to report dizziness?

Medicine uses placebos in two ways. One, they serve as controls in randomized, controlled trials. In a scientific trial, a placebo is a pill made to look identical to the research pill but contains only inactive ingredients. The placebo is given to the control group in a double-blind manner. That is, neither the researcher nor the subject knows whether they are receiving the active therapy or the inactive substitute. When a placebo serves in this manner, the British term "dummy" is less confusing.

The reason for these elaborate precautions is the placebo effect. This effect refers to the symptomatic improvement in some patients when they are given a dummy medication. Reasons for this effect are sophisticated. These may include the patient's hope for the new wonder drug, the careful attention of a caring doctor, or simply the disease's natural history. In any case, a dummy drug helps account for this effect. The tested research drug must outperform the placebo to be credited with a real therapeutic effect.

Confounding our understanding of the placebo is the natural history of diseases. Since most conditions can improve, at least temporarily, it is often impossible to determine how much of the observed improvement with dummy pills is due to the placebo effect. Or how much improvement represents the natural history of the disease. The process of enrolling patients in a trial, even in a nontreatment arm, involves recruitment of the patient (i.e., recognition). A complete explanation of the research trial occurs (i.e., attention). It involves making a correct diagnosis (i.e., reassurance). Blood tests are drawn (i.e., care). All these foregoing activities have a placebo effect by themselves.

Interest in the placebo effect became evident in the period 1935–1950. This effect explains why testimonials are not helpful in providing knowledge. The so-called commonsense idea that "I took this red pill and it cured my cold" is deceptive.

If there were no placebo effect, and if the natural history of a disease were perfectly understood, there would be no need for randomized-controlled trials. These controlled trials are explained in more detail in subsequent chapters, but briefly, the method consists of maneuvers to ensure a real therapeutic gain. A control group with the same disease takes a placebo. By doing so, the control group helps account for the natural history of the disease and the placebo effect. The control and treatment groups are chosen by chance (i.e., randomization), and the study is done without the patient or the evaluating physician knowing which patients are getting the active medicine (i.e., double-blind).

HISTORICAL ANTECEDENTS

The alternative view during the first few decades of the twentieth century was that astute physicians devoted to specializing in particular diseases could make judgments of the efficacy of treatment over the placebo effect. Studies have shown how easily even specialists can be mistaken. If a doctor that has devoted their life to understanding a particular disease can be misled, how much more the ill layperson who desperately wants to get better?

Before the twentieth century, the history of medical therapeutics could be called the era of the placebo effect, when there were few effective drugs apart from this salutary effect. Even into the twentieth century, patients continued to submit to purging, vomiting, poisoning, cutting, cupping, blistering, bleeding, freezing, heating, sweating, leeching, and shocking. Catharsis was a common theme for most treatments until the beginning of the twentieth century. Catharsis involved the removal of corrupt, evil humor or disease. Reviewing historical therapies, Shapiro says in summary:

> What useful drugs did exist (throughout history) were often used inappropriately, in inappropriate dosages, for scores of conditions, and physicians lacked the capacity to evaluate their usefulness, thus contributing to the loss of the benefit of these drugs for future generations. Despite this, historians continue to exaggerate the effectiveness of primitive medicine, without regard to its proven usefulness. The only resolution to the question of the efficacy of ancient drugs is to accurately determine the putative name of each ancient drug, its chemistry and methods of preparation, how it was used, and for what illnesses; to translate this information into current pharmacological knowledge; and to conduct in-vitro and in-vivo clinically controlled studies—a task not likely to be done anytime soon. Without such proof, the claims about the efficacy of ancient remedies have yet to be proved.[8]

There were, of course, a few isolated exceptions to the rule that historical drugs before the twentieth century were only placebos. Examples of effective treatments in history are cinchona bark and foxglove. These latter plants were later refined as quinine for malaria and digitalis for heart failure.

This view is strengthened by the fact that life expectancy has only recently changed throughout history. Moreover, there was no difference in longevity between geographical areas or between diverse cultures or medical practices. In other words, if we had effective therapies earlier in history, why didn't human survival improve over the millennia-old life expectancy average of 35–40 years? Longevity began to improve only in the West in the nineteenth century, and then in other parts of the world as the twentieth century progressed. Life expectancy in any given area only improved with the introduction of scientific medicine. The age at which a person dies is the strongest endpoint that cannot be driven by the patient or researcher. This is what researchers call a "hard endpoint" in long-term studies.

NOCEBO

Inert pills can also cause negative effects. The agent that does so is called a nocebo, and its result is called a nocebo effect. Beecher lists many toxic effects of placebos: fatigue 18%, headache 25%, nausea 10%, difficulty concentrating 15%.[9] And if the side effects are greater than the positive improvement, it defines the agent as a nocebo. The case cited at the beginning of this chapter was actually an example of a nocebo effect, rather than the more familiar placebo construct.

In another way, the nocebo effect can occur with negative expectations (something a caring physician would never intend). In an early experiment, an allergy sufferer was set to wheezing when shown an artificial rose. In another investigation, college students were told they might get a headache when a small electric current was passed through their heads. Two-thirds of the students reported headaches, even though no electric current was actually used.[10]

Thus, placebos can have positive and negative effects.

BE THE FIRST TO USE A MEDICINE

There is a recurrent theme in the history of treatments for angina pectoris or any other medical disease. When a new medicine is first introduced, there is general enthusiasm and hope for its effectiveness. In early studies and anecdotal reports, proponents of a new therapy are called "enthusiasts"; these enthusiasts report remarkable benefits in most patients.[11] Early non-blinded trials fail to control the placebo effect evoked by the investigator's enthusiastic expectations of success.

Later, skeptical investigators perform more adequately controlled trials. These doubting researchers tend to operate under circumstances that minimize the placebo effect and find the therapy no better than dummy pills. Negative reports continue to emanate, and the "new" therapy is abandoned with rapid disappearance from the medical literature.

This pattern is consistent: initial reports by the enthusiasts cite 70%–90% effectiveness, which falls to 30%–40% effectiveness, on the level with placebos, when the skeptics finish reporting.

This pattern has been so well-known that a nineteenth-century French physician, Armand Trousseau, joked, "You should treat as many patients as possible with the new drugs while they yet have the power to heal."

Placebos act rapidly. Relief of symptoms, principally pain, occurs within minutes to hours. The duration of relief is often cited as long as three months. However, there are records of prolonged pain relief lasting months and years. In trials for angina and rheumatoid arthritis, placebo effects have been shown to continue for as long as 30 months.[12]

There are other observed characteristics of the placebo effect. A large pill is more effective than a small pill. Blue-colored pills work better for anxiety, and red-colored pills work better for pain. A placebo given by injection is more powerful than a pill given by mouth. A dummy pill administered by a doctor appears more powerful than that given by a nurse or clerk. A placebo (or any medicine) sent in the mail, without human interaction, is the least effective. In trials, the more frequently the patient sees the physician during the study period, the greater the placebo effect. Furthermore, the more attention paid to a patient when he first visits the doctor for a symptom, the more satisfactory will be the result.[12]

It has also been shown that patients are more likely to experience a placebo effect if they like and have confidence in their doctor and if treatment is prescribed enthusiastically. "The doctor who fails to have a placebo effect on his patients should become a pathologist."[12]

HOW DO PLACEBOS WORK?

The author wants to make clear that we are not discussing the idea of suggestibility here. The placebo effect is not a hypnotic idea planted into the weak-willed patient in some mysterious way against their inclination. How might a placebo work, if not by suggestion to the weak-minded?

In a landmark study, Dr. Levine was the first to report on the induction of internally made narcotic-like molecules (i.e., endorphins) in the body in response to a placebo after surgery.[13] Patients were studied after extraction of impacted third molars removed under nitrous oxide anesthesia, and a short-acting local nerve block (both of these pain relievers would be dissipated within one to two hours). Three to four hours after extraction, some patients were given placebo injections in a double-blind fashion. If they responded with pain reduction, they were then given, without their knowledge, a drug called naloxone, which completely reversed the pain relief achieved with the previously given placebo.

Naloxone is a medicine known as a specific reversal agent of the effect of narcotics, opioids, and endorphins. Naloxone binds to pain relief receptors in the body more tightly than its competitors. However, it does not activate the receptor to provide pain relief. It is like putting the wrong key into a lock. The lock cannot be opened, but neither can the proper key gain entrance as long as the wrong key is jammed into the lock. Consequently, the pain-relieving effects of the endorphin or narcotic molecules disappear.

Returning to our dental example, the human body can produce its own narcotic molecules known as endorphins. These molecules are recruited when the body encounters pain and anticipates relief with a placebo. When reversal of placebo achieved pain occurs, this provides proof of at least one biochemical mechanism for the placebo effect. The endorphin response to placebo has been shown in many studies. Endorphins are only part of the story, as the response to placebo is a complex reaction.

Much effort has been devoted to distinguishing the characteristics that would help identify placebo responders. The consensus is that different parameters of age, gender, education, etc., do not predict who will respond with improved symptoms. As Thompson puts it, "The notion that only some of us have such a 'weakness' is absurd."[14] Nevertheless, the placebo response for any given person varies from time to time, and from situation to situation. The same subject may have a placebo response during one trial, but not in a subsequent trial.

Many reviewers of the placebo effect agree that the inert pills relieve only illness and do not change the course of disease. Illness is the experience of the patient. It is what the patient perceives is taking place. This includes his or her symptoms. In contrast, a disease is a change in body structure that the doctor can see on X-ray, biopsy, or surgery.

However, if pain disappears with the placebo, many laymen conclude the disease has been helped. Steve McQueen, for example, reported to the world that his visits to unorthodox treatment clinics in Mexico made him pain-free and that his cancer (mesothelioma—a rare lung cancer) was therefore getting better. Unfortunately, two months later he died of cancer.[15]

The author realizes he is belaboring the point, but this distinction is crucial. So often, after a layman encounters talk about the placebo effect, he or she will ask why we don't use these inexpensive pills for their beneficial effect.

Hopefully, the reader will avoid the latter misunderstanding in the following published correspondence:

My name is. ...I live in Cali, Columbia. A few days ago I listened about placebo effect. My father has cancer, and I believe a placebo can help him. I need to know where I can get the sugar pills or saline injections, and how I must give to him. My father's doctors have said his cancer is very bad, and it's so difficult to treat. He has been following a treatment since 8 years, but he always fall ill again. I think the placebo is his last hope. If you can help me, I'll be grateful all my life.[16]

If the reader expects a placebo will help this cancer patient, they have missed the point of the discussion of illness versus disease. Assuming an efficacious treatment is impossible, he will be better served with comforting care, truth, and appropriate pain management. Successful pain management is alleviation of most of the pain while allowing the patient to stay clear-minded with a normal sleep pattern. A palliative approach would give predictable relief compared to the uncertainty of placebo.

IMPURE PLACEBO

Modern physicians rarely use placebos outside of clinical research. Yet, what is often done is to give a pill with proven therapeutic benefit for another disease, but which has none for the one prescribed. An example would be an antibiotic prescription for viral upper respiratory infections. Antibiotics do not work against viruses. Many patients demand an antibiotic from their doctor, who often oblige for fear of losing business.

There are other examples, like giving an antiulcer drug to patients with no ulcer, but who continue to complain of upset stomach. If a patient with one disease receives a pill proven only effective in another disease, then the pill is an impure placebo. Physicians who would be horrified to give pure placebos often give impure placebos.

CONCLUSION

The placebo effect is a complex therapeutic influence that arises from expectation and conditioning. One that elicits symptomatic relief. This effect is immediate and usually abates in the short term but can last for years. There is no convincing evidence that this reduction of symptoms changes the physical disease in any way. Simply put, placebos do not help people live longer. For thousands of years, until smallpox vaccination began in earnest in the nineteenth century, the life span of human beings was unchanged worldwide. This is proof that addressing symptoms alone does little to prolong the length of life.

In research, the placebo arm helps control and separate all factors in the non-treated group that could affect the outcome. Controlling for the placebo effect is a cornerstone of modern scientific medicine.

The doctor in his or her being has prodigious power to help people feel better. A confident manner in diagnosis, explanation, and expectation of treatment benefit, along with a caring manner, provide a powerful effect for good, even if it is a placebo. When combined with medicines proven to have a disease-modifying effect, the patient can experience the best of both worlds.

NOTES

1   Benson H, McCallie Jr DP. Angina pectoris and the placebo effect. *New England Journal of Medicine* 1979;300; pp. 1424–9.

2   Dimond EG, Kittle CF, Crockett JE. Comparison of internal mammary artery ligation and sham operation for angina pectoris. *American Journal of Cardiology* 1960;5; pp. 483–6.

3   Cobb LA, Thomas GI, Dillard DH, Merendino KA, Bruce RA. An evaluation of internal-mammary-artery ligation by a double-blind technique. *New England Journal of Medicine* 1959;260; pp. 1115–8.

4 Alda A. *The Wonder Pill*. Alexandria, VA: PBS Home Video; 2003.

5 Moseley JB, O'Malley K, Petersen NJ, et al. A controlled trial of arthroscopic surgery for osteoarthritis of the knee. *New England Journal of Medicine* 2002;347; pp. 81–8. DOI: 10.1056/NEJMoa013259

6 Felson DT, Buckwalter J. Debridement and lavage for osteoarthritis of the knee. *New England Journal Medicine* 2002;347; pp. 132–3. DOI: 10.1056/NEJMoa013259

7 Thompson WG. *The Placebo Effect and Health: Combining Science and Compassionate Care*. Amheerst, NY: Prometheus Books; 2005, p. 138.

8 Shapiro AK, Shapiro E. *The Powerful Placebo: From Ancient Priest to Modern Physician*. Baltimore: Johns Hopkins University Press; 1997, p. 229.

9 Beecher HK. The powerful placebo. *Journal of the American Medical Association* 1955;159; pp. 1602–6.

10 Ehrlich R. *Eight Preposterous Propositions*. Princeton, NJ: Princeton University Press; 2003.

11 Beecher HK. Surgery as placebo: A quantitative study of bias. *JAMA* 1961;176; pp. 1102–7.

12 Thompson, pp. 40–9.

13 Levine J, Gordon N, Fields H. The mechanism of placebo analgesia. *Lancet* 1978;312; pp. 654–7.

14 Thompson, p. 201.

15 Buckman R. *Feeling Better, Getting Better?* Princeton, NJ: Films for the Humanities and Sciences; 2001.

16 Guess HA, Kleinman A, Kusek JW, Engel LW. *The Science of the Placebo: Toward an Interdisciplinary Research Agenda*. London: BMJ Books; 2002, p. 36.

14 John Brinkley and Goat Gland Transplantation

"A man is as old as his glands" and "all energy is sex energy" were two favorite advertising phrases that John Brinkley, pretend physician, boomed over his Kansas radio station in the 1920s.[1] At his clinic in Milford, Kansas, he transplanted live donor goat glands (testicles) onto men's native testicles. His was a siren call to men that feared they were losing their grip on manhood. This miracle was done for the "bargain price" of $750 (no credit, please).

Dr. Brinkley noted,

> Contrast the castrated animal, of any species, with the natural male or female. Note the difference, for instance, between the stallion and gelding. The former stands erect, neck arched, mane flowing, champing the bit, stamping the ground, seeking the female, while the gelding stands around half asleep, cowardly and listless, going into action only when goaded, with no interest in anything.[2]

Who was this dubious physician, shameless radio promoter, and self-proclaimed martyr? John Romulus Brinkley claimed to have graduated in 1902 from a one-room rural high school in North Carolina. At age 22, he married his first wife, Sally Wike, and moved to Chicago. Despite not having gone to college, he was accepted into Bennett Medical College, an eclectic school, not approved by the American Medical Association (AMA).[3] In a biography authorized by Brinkley, Wood claims the aspiring doctor worked so hard the next three years in medical school that he once collapsed in the classroom from exhaustion.[4] The stress of work and school led to ruin. His wife left him, and he dropped out of medical school.

Under oath, later in life, Brinkley maintained he attended the college department of the National University of Arts and Sciences at St. Louis, Missouri, from September 1911 to June 1913. The school was well-known as a diploma mill, as long as the buyer had $100. The parchment issued by the dean of the school, W.P. Sachs, states, "John R. Brinkley has completed two years of college work at the National University of Arts and Sciences and appeared before me and in a written examination…has made passing grades…entitling to the credits annexed." Sachs later admitted under oath the paper was fraudulent and was issued for cash consideration.

Newspaper accounts in 1913 have a man named J. R. Brinkley operating as an "Electro Medic Doctor" in Greenville, South Carolina, where he and a partner advertised, "Are You a Manly Man Full of Vigor?" Apparently, many Greenville males worried about the answer to this question and flocked to the clinic where they would receive an injection of salvarsan (the accepted anti-syphilitic treatment) for $25. But it was only a solution of colored distilled water. Sensing their scam disintegrating, Brinkley and his partner skipped town with unpaid bills.[5]

As Brinkley fled Greenville, he traveled through Memphis, Tennessee, and met a woman named Minnie Jones. After a whirlwind courtship, John married her on August 23, 1913. He neglected to tell Minnie he was still married. Brinkley was later arrested in Tennessee, charged with fraud in Greenville, and extradited back to South Carolina. The charges were dropped after his father-in-law, Dr. Tiberius Jones, paid the creditors.

In any case, in 1915, Brinkley got a break. He found that the Eclectic Medical School of Kansas City, an institution also not accredited by the AMA, would accept his previous medical school credits. Wood relates that Brinkley's credits from Bennett were granted on the basis of Brinkley's testimony.[6] With his past credits expeditiously taken care of, the Eclectic Medical School allowed him to

DOI: 10.1201/9781003324058-14

finish his degree in one year for $100. Young Brinkley matriculated and, by his account, finished his coursework in a few weeks.

Finally, John had a "diploma" and a "medical degree." Unfortunately, the licensing boards of Kansas and 39 other states did not recognize his alma mater. In response, the head of the Eclectic University gathered the entire graduating class of 1915 and headed south to Arkansas, where the school was recognized. After a two-and-a-half day examination from the Eclectic Medical Examining Board of Arkansas, Brinkley apparently passed the test and received his license.[7]

Brinkley answered an advertisement for a position in Milford, Kansas. He sensed opportunity in a town only ten miles from the geographical center of the lower 48 states. Brinkley was under the mistaken impression that the town had a population of 2,000. Arriving, he found a tiny hamlet of 200 inhabitants. In 1917, Milford Kansas was the prototypic town of American rural humor. There were no traffic problems; the roads weren't paved; it did not have electric lights. There was no running water unless one ran to the well with a bucket. The railroad depot was a mile from town, in the middle of a cornfield. The town drugstore was empty. Brinkley rented the pharmacy for $8 a month and put in a stock of patent medicines.

BRINKLEY AND THE BILLY GOAT

In his general practice, Brinkley noted measles, whooping cough, and hernias. Then, two weeks after starting work, on the so-called Day of Discovery, Brinkley describes meeting a farmer late one night in his backroom. Mr. "X's" (as Wood's biography identifies him) self-diagnosis was, "All done in. No pep." The farmer pleaded with the young eclectic doctor to do something. The patient confessed to being a "flat tire." The doctor could not help, and the conversation became general. The news topic of the day was glandular transplantation. Referring to the farmer's knowledge of livestock, Brinkley observed, "You must have seen just what I have seen—those rams and buck goats." The doctor laughed, "You wouldn't have any trouble if you had a pair of those buck glands in you."

"Well, why don't you put 'em in?"

Brinkley rejected the suggestion offhand. He told the patient that it was biologically impossible for the organ of a lower animal to be transplanted into a higher member of the animal kingdom.[5] Brinkley eventually relented and performed the operation. But he felt uneasy about the whole affair. However,

[Brinkley] could reassure himself that the deed was done in seclusion, and the situation carried with it built in protection. The patient was not likely to broadcast that he had tried to pep up his sex life—and failed.[1]

The patient reported the return of normal libido, and a year later, Dr. Brinkley delivered a baby boy to the patient's wife. The parents named the boy "Billy," in recognition of the role of the donor in his father's re-treading operation.

While the first patient paid Dr. Brinkley $150, the standard charge eventually became $750 or more.[8] Charges included, if the transplant recipient were inclined, a stroll among the frisky bucks to select his lusty donor in advance. Minnie then procured the testicular glands from the young goat.[9] Using local anesthesia, Dr. Brinkley inserted the goat glands under the scrotal skin of the patient. The operation took 15 minutes.

GOAT AND MONKEY GLANDS

To put the Goat Gland Doctor in his times, newspaper reports and gossip columns of the 1920s often were about (European) doctors performing monkey gland (testicular) transplantation. There were monkey gland jokes and monkey gland novels. Stage plays about this dubious operation often were flippant, and the sexual connotations underscored. Critics of the gland operation were accused of "prudery."

Despite a series of surgical studies in animals, published from 1929 to 1931, that failed to show any favorable effect of the operation, Hamilton writes, "[P]ublic disenchantment with human testicle transplantation was slow, as if many wanted to believe that rejuvenation was possible."[10]

VISITING BRINKLEY'S HOSPITAL

What was it like for a patient to visit the hospital in Milford? John Zahner, a Lenexa, Kansas farmer, described his trip to the reporter from the Kansas City Star:

"For a year, I sat here every evening and listened to Dr. Brinkley talk over the radio. I am 64 years old and have prostate trouble, and Dr. Brinkley described my symptoms and sufferings exactly, and he kept telling over and over again how he could cure all such cases. I naturally thought he must be all he claimed he was, for I could not conceive it to be possible that this great government of ours would give a license to a quack and charlatan to operate a radio broadcasting station with which to rope in victims. I had read of the federal radio commission and how careful it was to protect the public from frauds, and Dr. Brinkley himself used to emphasize over the radio that if were not all he claimed he was, the government would soon put him off the air, and I reasoned it must be so.

Well, I wrote to Dr. Brinkley, and then the letters from him began to pour in on me, urging me to come for an examination anyway. Finally, a date was set. ... We were met at the train in Milford and taken to the hospital, arriving there at 4 o'clock Sunday afternoon. I was the second man to be examined by Dr. Osborn.[11] I did not see Brinkley. Osborn pretended to x-ray me, and he jabbed an instrument into me that made me bleed. He said my prostate gland was as big as his fist [e.g., a normal prostate gland would be the size of a walnut]. I was sent to bed, and all night long, until 4 o'clock the next morning, those men were being examined, one after the other, each being frightened and sent to bed.

Sometime after midnight, Mrs. Brinkley came and said to me: 'You have a bad case of prostate trouble.' She called it a 'borderline case' and I understood that meant that I was close to the borderline that separates life from death. She insisted that I must be operated upon at once. I might not live to get home unless I did. She scared me. She guaranteed me that in three days after the operation, I would have relief. She had a check all filled out for me to sign. It was for $750. I believe I would have never signed it had she come to me in daylight, but at that uncanny hour of night, with sick men all limping up and down the halls, lights flickering, examinations going on, I was unduly influenced and I signed it.

That morning, at 9 o'clock, Dr. Osborn operated on me. I was in bed only half a day. On Friday, Dr. Brinkley came to my room, the first time I had seen him, and I said to him,

'Doctor, I am five times as bad as when I came.'

'That's natural and to be expected; it will be a year before you are fully well,' he said.

'But they told me I would be well in three days. Your wife told me that,' I insisted.

'You must have misunderstood her; yours is a borderline case, and you may have to come back for another operation later on,' he said. I was given notice that I must leave Saturday, and all the patients who had gone there with me were cleared out before Sunday. That is the way they operate. They get patients to come in batches each Sunday and clear them all out before the following Sunday, when a new batch comes in. In my opinion, that is done so the newcomers will not have a chance to talk to those who have been operated on. ... After I got home, it began to dawn on me that I had been victimized and I tried to stop payment on the check I had given, but Brinkley had already cashed it, and its payment was guaranteed and my bank told me I might as well pay it as I would be sued on it and it could be collected. I borrowed the money to pay it."[12]

The reader can rest assured this operation did not increase the secretion of male hormones or any other so-called vital substance. As one journal editor criticized, testis-grafting was "nothing more or less than a piece of dead meat put in the wrong place."[10]

Indeed, in Brinkley's famous libel trial of 1938, Brinkley admitted that a "majority" of the goat glands were gradually "absorbed" by the patients' bodies.[13] Further evidence the operation was hocus-pocus turns on the idea that Brinkley abandoned his operation in 1933. He claimed commercial glandular preparations could be used just as well. And the commercial tissue could be injected intravenously. Still, when these ampules for injection were later taken by some patients for chemical analysis, it was noted they contained distilled water and methylene blue, a blue ink.[14]

What would account for the dramatic improvement male patients claimed from his operation? Certainly, the placebo effect, described in a prior chapter, would be operant here. A surgical placebo is much stronger than a medical placebo. Much of male impotency is caused by performance anxiety. If this apprehension can be lowered, subsequent relaxation ameliorates the impotency. The patient's belief that recovery would occur, and their knowledge of the success of other patients, would prove a powerful aphrodisiac—that is, until an adverse life experience again raised anxiety.

As the Goat Gland Doctor's fame increased, he became the "butt" of jokes— "What is the fastest four-legged animal in the world? Answer: a billy goat going past the Brinkley hospital." Or, when Brinkley flew overhead in his plane, the farmer's daughter would explain to her aging father, "Pa, Doc Brinkley is coming after you."[5]

BRINKLEY IMITATES A DOCTOR

Brinkley knew he needed to look like a doctor. With his retreating hairline, personality glasses, tufted goatee, and a wisp of a mustache, along with a grave and magisterial manner, he looked every inch the physician (Figure 14.1).

The wall in Dr. Brinkley's office displayed many certificates: BA, MD, LL.D, ScD, PhD, DPH, Chief Surgeon, College of Physicians and Surgeons (strictly his own institution), head of Brinkley Laboratories, and member of the National Geographic Society. The only valid one was likely the dues paying membership of the National Geographic. Society (see note 15).

Brinkley eventually decided to hire an advertising consultant to help him get the news out about his operation. As news spread, he began to attract well-known personalities to the tiny town. Dr. Tobias, chancellor of the Chicago Law School, underwent the Brinkley operation and reported remarkable success. "I left the hospital feeling 25 years younger," he told newspaper reporters. In a photographic pose of a boxer in the ring, he continued, "and I seem to grow still

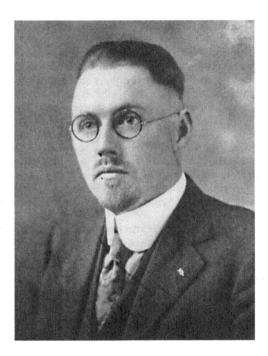

Figure 14.1 John R. Brinkley, Circa 1921. (From Kansas State Historical Society. Public Domain.)

younger every day!" The chancellor introduced him to other famous people, many of whom underwent his operation.[2]

BRINKLEY AND RADIO

Inspired by a radio station he noticed while on a trip in California, Brinkley returned to Kansas and, in September 1923, opened up the fourth radio station in Kansas and the first in Kansas to receive an Federal Communications Commission license. The call letters were KFKB, for which Brinkley said stood for "Kansas First, Kansas Best." Brinkley refused to use phonograph records and promoted local amateur talent to build one of the largest radio audiences in America at the time.

Brinkley used the radio station for what he called a Medical Question Box. Brinkley gave the Medical Question Box three times a day to answer questions sent to him in the mail. For example, he would read the symptoms of "A. B. of Garden City" over the air and end up prescribing preparations "C, D, and E" for this patient. He told this person and others with the same complaint to order these. Soon, Brinkley filled a huge amount of prescriptions from his store, and this seriously depleted the business of other druggists, especially those in the surrounding states.

This led to a delegation of perturbed pharmacists visiting the Milford doctor. They presented their complaint that his mail-order business was ruining theirs. Brinkley worked with them in a two-hour session on the plans for the "Brinkley Pharmaceutical Association," which would include 500 pharmacies in Kansas and surrounding states.

To avoid the possibility of his listeners becoming confused with technical terms, Brinkley returned to the nineteenth-century patent era system of giving a number to prescriptions. Then, Brinkley would prescribe by number and the listener could go to the associated pharmacy and ask for the Brinkley number to get the intended medication. What the numbers stood for was a secret Brinkley instructed his pharmacists to keep in their safe. Brinkley was to get one dollar kickback for every prescription thus sold. Most prescriptions were about $3.00 for generic items, such as aspirin or castor oil, which, if known, would usually sell for less than $1.00. As Brinkley raked in the money, the associated Brinkley pharmacies noted a dramatic increase in sales to as much as $100 or more a day.

An example of what the radio listeners would hear after the pharmaceutical association was formed would be as follows: "This little lady has been seeing spots before her eyes, has dizzy spells, and is constipated. Prescriptions 66 and 74, which she can procure at the Acme Drugstore in..., at $5 and $7, will bring her relief."[16]

Needless to say, this type of brazen and dangerous practice of medicine (i.e., without seeing the patient) led to a marked diminution of business in the pharmacies that were not part of his association.

BRINKLEY'S WEALTH

Brinkley's annual income in the late 1920s consisted of the prescription business bringing in anywhere from $400,000 to $750,000 per year. If he performed the operations per week, as he claimed for 40 weeks annually (he had three months' vacation in the summer), his surgical income would have been $1.5 million per year for around $2 million per annum.[16] In contrast, the average physician was making $3,000 to $5,000 per year.

Brinkley's practice overhead had to be substantial, so we do not know what his net income was, but his lifestyle was ostentatious and even gaudy. As evidence of his luxurious lifestyle, he was driving up to a dozen luxury cars ($7,000 apiece for Lincolns or 16-cylinder Cadillacs); one of his Cadillacs had "Dr. Brinkley" or "JRB" emblazoned in gold plates in 13 places.[16] He also went through three expensive yachts. His last yacht was 171 feet in length, cost $500,000, and required a 21-man crew to operate.

He and his wife had a penchant for diamonds and owned some the size of hazelnuts. John had an 11-carat diamond on his right hand and a 14 carat on his left. His tie pin contained a 24-carat diamond. The total value of the jewels the Brinkleys were decked out in was estimated to be greater than $100,000. In addition to these possessions, they had a 12-passenger, twin-engine airplane costing $58,000, to which he added $20,000 of improvements.

The contrast with the economic hardships of most Kansans in the late '20s could not be starker. Things only worsened when the Wall Street crash occurred in 1929, but this did not seem to dent Brinkley's economic activity.

In public, Brinkley alleged he was trying to be scientific. Brinkley declared he had attempted to report the technique of his operation and findings to the *Journal of the American Medical Association*. The editor of the journal, Maurice Fishbein, denied ever receiving any submission. Brinkley later declared he had received a letter back from the editor of the *Journal of the American Medical Association* (*JAMA*) saying the journal could not publish such "non-descript" material.[1] Brinkley also alleged he sought other journals without success.

Despite all his money, Brinkley did not persevere in publishing the details of his operation for medical peer review. He hired consultants to tell him how to do everything else managing his practice and money. He authored books for laymen about his operation but made no effort to hire people that could tell him how to report his results in a publishable manner, which would enable his scientific peers to evaluate his results.

"PERSECUTION" RAMPS UP

The campaign by the Kansas State Medical Board and the AMA against Brinkley needs to be put into historical perspective. At the beginning of the twentieth century, the quality of American medical schools was very uneven. There were a few excellent medical schools associated with top-notch universities on the one hand, and many so-called proprietary schools that had libraries without books, nonexistent laboratories, and faculty too preoccupied with their private practices to do justice to their teaching responsibilities.

The highly critical *Flexner Report* in 1910 described the woeful quality of most American medical schools. The *Flexner Report*, supported by the private Carnegie Foundation, shamed the medical profession into imposing higher standards for its schools. Its principal recommendation was that all medical schools be tied to a university. This spelled doom for all proprietary schools. Numbers tell the story. In 1906, there were 162 medical schools; by 1915, this had dropped to 95. The next step for the AMA was to police the state licensure systems. This weeded out the "very worst" doctors who had graduated from the defunct schools. State after state began forcing eclectics and homeopaths to conform to the new standards or find other work.

Morris Fishbein became editor of *JAMA* in September 1924. Fishbein became an energetic advocate of the association's interests both through its publication and as a speaker. He published several articles in *JAMA* that were critical of John Brinkley and other quack doctors. By 1928, Fishbein and his associates at the AMA had monitored Brinkley's unorthodox methods for years but had taken little action. Fishbein wrote,

> As long as he confined himself to goat gland practice, we didn't bother much about him, but when he began prescribing over the radio for the ills of patients he had never seen, treating dangerous afflictions by air, some agency simply had to come to the front for the protection of the public.

Then, in early 1930, A. B. McDonald, a reporter for the *Kansas City Star*, joined the anti-Brinkley campaign.[17] The *Star* printed vivid stories of Brinkley's fits of insobriety, cursing, and rage, told by disgruntled patients and hospital employees. A former head nurse told the *Star* how Brinkley privately ridiculed his own ideas and mocked patients gullible enough to have his operation done as "old fools."[18]

McDonald interviewed Brinkley and reviewed his operation. His series included many death certificates for Brinkley patients that had died after the operation. Later, in the legal suit, Brinkley responded to questions about each of the death certificates he signed over the years. Under cross-examination, he recounted what he believed each one had died of. He denied any were the result of the operation. Yet, without a third party doing an autopsy, all such descriptions by Brinkley were of course suspect.

On April 10, 1930, Fishbein turned up the heat in the anti-Brinkley campaign with an editorial in the AMA journal calling Brinkley "a charlatan of the rankest sort" and urged the Federal Radio Commission (FRC) to consider pulling his radio license. On April 29, 1930, Dr. L.F. Barney, president of the Kansas Medical Society, filed a formal complaint with the Kansas Board of Medical Registration, requesting it revoke Brinkley's license.

Brinkley did not stand still. He filed a $5 million lawsuit for libel against the *Kansas City Star*, and a $600,000 damage suit against Morris Fishbein for authoring the quack article. Also, Brinkley fought back on his radio station, referring to the AMA as the "Amateur Meatcutters Association" and Morris Fishbein as "Little Old Fishy." Minnie Brinkley referred to Fishbein as the "poor Jew-boy." Brinkley, referring to the AMA, also said, "These M.D.'s are a stealing, thieving, lying bunch," in one 1930 broadcast. "I'll grind their heads off under my heel like I would a snake." He cast himself as a martyr who was being steamrolled by a monopoly. They were out to ruin him because of "jealousy" over his success. He predicted to the AMA, "I will beat you because I have right and truth, and these will eventually triumph."

Brinkley allowed his suit against Fishbein to lapse in February 1934, when he declined to pay $1,000 in additional court costs. He also quietly dropped his libel suit against the *Kansas City Star*.

The year 1930 would see tremendous publicity in the coverage of the Brinkley hearings before the FRC and the Kansas Medical Board. Sex, quackery, and politics all rolled into one created enormous interest. According to Lee, nothing like these hearings had ever happened in the medical profession, either in Kansas or nationally.[5]

The hearings proved entertaining. But in the end, on June 13, 1930, the FRC, by a vote of three to two, declined to renew Brinkley's KFKB radio license. Outraged, Brinkley charged that the AMA and even President Hoover were part of a conspiracy against him.[19] KFKB continued to broadcast throughout the fall, pending an appeal to the US Supreme Court. When the Supreme Court refused to hear the case, Brinkley closed up and sold the station.

With KFKB lost, Brinkley went reeling a month later into hearings before the State Medical Board in Topeka. It seems evident that toward the end of the hearings, Brinkley felt things were not going well for him. In summation, the Goat Gland Doctor announced what he felt would be a positive clincher. He challenged the board representatives to watch him do his surgery in Milford.

A delegation of 12 doctors was soon dispatched to visit Brinkley's hospital in Milford. They dutifully watched him operate. After the operations, Brinkley told his biographer that "the doctors left with their heads hung in shame, with their tails between their legs liked whipped curs." Not quite. The *Kansas City Star* reported the doctors saying Mrs. Brinkley's method of procuring the glands was unscientific and potentially unsterile. They felt there was a danger the glands were contaminated with tetanus germs. In any case, the Kansas State Medical Board soon revoked Dr. Brinkley's medical license.

ESCAPING THE FEDERAL TRADE COMMISSION WITH MEXICAN RADIO

In the midst of these troubles, Brinkley was invited by the city of Del Rio, Texas, to move his clinic to the Rio Grande location. As he considered moving from Kansas to Texas, two of his Milford doctors decamped with Brinkley's list of patients and prospects, along with the secretary responsible for the panel.

Moving to Del Rio, Brinkley created the most powerful radio station in the United States with the call letters XER. By virtue of its location on the Mexican side of the Rio Grande, XER could boom to the entire United States and evade regulation by the FRC. Remote control lines from his studio in Del Rio crossed the Rio Grande to XER, which allowed him to broadcast from the United States.

He converted a six-story Del Rio hotel into the new Brinkley hospital and built a $200,000 mansion under the shadows of XER's transmitting towers. While Brinkley was back in business, his hospital no longer advertised the standard goat gland transplant that had made him famous. The former operation was unnecessary, he professed, because newly invented glandular emulsions offered the same benefits from a simple injection. This more effective solution, as mentioned earlier, was a worthless combination of distilled water and a blue dye.

Brinkley continued to boom his medical advice over the airwaves. Sometimes, this transmitter was the most powerful transmitter in North America. And, while Brinkley did not exert as close control over programming at XER as he had at KFKB, outlandish things occurred from people that rented time on his radio station. All the performers on any station were rated by how much mail they could "pull." Rose Dawn, Brinkley's personal astrologer, became one of the most effective mail pullers in radio history. She would read listeners' horoscopes or give lovelorn advice for $1 per service.

THE NOOSE TIGHTENS

In the midst of the Great Depression, Brinkley made more than a million dollars in 1936 and 1937. However, in January and February 1938, two negative articles appeared in a journal called *Hygeia*. These were written by Dr. Morris Fishbein. Brinkley felt they were the cause of his income in 1939 going down to $810,000. Brinkley sued. It was recognized that the requested compensation of $250,000 was not what the libel lawsuit was based upon. The man that wore a fortune in jewelry on his person would be the happiest man in the country if he got a one-cent verdict as vindication over Dr. Fishbein.

When the trial began in a Del Rio, Texas, courtroom in March 1939, Brinkley felt confident that a jury of local citizens would consider him one of their own. But Fishbein's lawyers turned the tables. They repeatedly pointed out Brinkley was not a common man, but one that wore a 14-carat diamond ring, owned a dozen automobiles, traveled the world on personal luxury liners he possessed, and even employed a private tutor for his 11-year-old son.

The income for physicians in the United States in the 1930s was about $5,000. Fishbein proclaimed, on the stand, that he knew of no other physicians that earned a gross income of over $1 million. "That's not medical practice, that's big business."

The jury deliberated for four hours and returned a favorable verdict for Morris Fishbein. Brinkley's attorneys appealed, but the circuit court in New Orleans concluded,

> There is no doubt whatever that the plaintiff by his methods violated acceptable standards of medical ethics—the plaintiff should be considered a charlatan and a quack in the ordinary, well-understood meaning of those words.[20]

The US Supreme Court denied further review. While Brinkley had been sued previously for malpractice, he had always managed to brazen through it or settle it out of court. But the Fishbein libel case officially and legally branded him a "quack" and "charlatan." As a result, wrongful death suits against him—claiming more than $3 million in damages—multiplied rapidly in the following year. In 1940, a dozen more suits were brought against him.

The numerous legal actions caused Brinkley to flee to a hotel in Memphis and direct his Arkansas hospital business from there, thus eluding Arkansas process servers. Nevertheless, he still paid $900,000 to settle three cases out of court. When Brinkley managed to stay out of the Arkansas courts by remaining in Tennessee, a federal judge was forced to award judgments against him by default. Word of Brinkley's legal troubles quickly spread across the country, and patients coming to his hospital slowed to a trickle.

As Brinkley's finances deteriorated, so did his health. Years of smoking and stress had taken a toll. Ironically, while he himself needed rejuvenation, the

Goat Gland Doctor did not undergo the operation. Following a heart attack, the 56-year-old John Brinkley died on May 26, 1941.

"[Brinkley] stood among tent-show medical quacks as an eagle among sparrows."[21] The dictionary defines quack and charlatan as applying to a person who unscrupulously pretends to knowledge or skill they do not possess. While these terms describe John Brinkley, perhaps con man would be better.

Brinkley clearly knew he was fraudulent when he administered blue water as an active medicine. His abandonment of goat gland transplantation also shows he concluded it did not work. Even if he started the operation in 1917 with a mistaken belief, his failure to repudiate it later tells us of his continuing intent to deceive. Brinkley could have easily determined how to report his operation to the peer-reviewed journals and other forums of the scientific community. But at every point, Brinkley declined to do so in favor of the so-called scientific (and uncritical) newspaper story.

Since the mid-1980s in America, we have discontinued the terms "quack" and "charlatan" in a fit of postmodern political correctness. In their place, we have taken up the banner of alternative and complementary medicine. However, what really exists is medicine that has been proven to work and that which is unproven or disproved. When promoters knowingly push untested or invalidated substances as effective, they need to be called quacks.

It may never be known what the real damages inflicted by Brinkley were. The charges for his operation were outlandish at a time when health insurance did not exist. How many Kansas family farms, struggling in the harsh economic conditions of the worst depression ever, were destroyed by gullible patients hoping for rejuvenation? Also, we must not forget the 6,000 goats that gave their all.

NOTES

1 Carson G. *The Roguish World of Doctor Brinkley*. New York: Rinehart; 1960, pp. 34–78.

2 Fowler G, Crawford B. *Border Radio: Quacks, Yodelers, Pitchmen, Psychics, and Other Amazing Broadcasters of the American Airwaves*. Revised Edition. Austin, TX: University of Texas Press; 2010, pp. 21–36.

3 Eclectic medicine was a philosophy that combined usage of herbal treatment with homeopathy (i.e., very tiny doses of medicine), which was active from roughly 1825 to 1939, when the last school of Eclectic treatment closed.

4 His biographer, Clement Wood, seems to have written only what Brinkley told him. Wood painted in *The Life of a Man* a picture of a backwoods boy growing up with experiences like Abraham Lincoln. Wood's biography is filled with known contradictions and misstatements of facts. Carson estimates Wood was paid $5,000 (about $50,000 now) for writing *The Life of a Man*.

5 Lee RA. *The Bizarre Careers of John R. Brinkley*. Lexington, KY: University Press of Kentucky; 2002, pp. 20–60.

6 Can the reader imagine getting medical school credit simply by telling a school how many courses you had allegedly taken somewhere else?

7 Four years later, the Eclectic School in Kansas City closed its doors after being implicated in a diploma-mill school scandal. But Brinkley was now a licensed doctor. He turned around and then used a common practice called

reciprocity, whereby he could obtain a license in Kansas, Tennessee, and Texas without having to pass another exam. Reciprocity between states for a medical license cannot be done today.

8   These costs need to be put in perspective. In the early 1920s, a model T Ford cost $400. Thus, the standard charge was nearly two times a new economy automobile!

9   The rest of the carcass was disposed of.

10 Hamilton D. *The Monkey Gland Affair*. London: Chatto & Windus; 1986, pp. 109–28.

11 Neither Dr. Osborn nor Mrs. Brinkley were ever licensed to practice medicine in Kansas and both had "diplomas" from schools that were involved in the diploma-mill scandals and subsequently closed.

12 Bureau of Investigation John R. Brinkley, Quack. The *Kansas City Star* helps turn on the light (excerpt from *Kansas City Star*) *Journal of the American Medical Association* 1930;94; pp. 1339–40. DOI: 10.1001/jama.1930.02710430063027

13 The author, who was board certified in liver transplantation, understands that a xenograft (meaning tissue from one species of animal to another) would have been immediately rejected and destroyed within a matter of a few hours to a few days. This assumes that the testicle was even viable even before transplanting it.

14 The billy goats certainly endorsed his chicanery.

15 Never has a man gone to school so little and come away with so many degrees! (BA means bachelor of arts or a graduate of a four-year college, MD means doctor of medicine or graduate of a medical school, LL.D means doctor of law degree in the United States, ScD means a doctor of science degree in the British Commonwealth (as opposed to the equivalent of PhD in the United States, meaning an advanced doctoral degree from any university department so qualified) [but of course he also listed a PhD after his name], and a DPH (doctor of public health).

16 Lee, pp. 79–80.

17 A.B. McDonald was a veteran reporter who, shortly after his Brinkley sequence, penned a series of articles that helped solve a murder case in Amarillo, Texas, leading to his winning a Pulitzer Prize.

18 Lee, p. 91.

19 Lee, p. 102.

20 Lee, p. 218.

21 Carson, front book cover.

15 Laetrile, Cyanide, and Ernst Krebs

> Just take three grams of laetrile per day in conjunction with our special "metabolic" diet, and you will control or eliminate active cancer in three weeks. If you don't have cancer yet, if you will just eat ten raw apricot kernels per day, this will prevent any development of cancer.[1,2]

These were the bizarre claims of a dangerous health cult. The cult originated with two men, each named Ernst T. Krebs, father and son. They brought laetrile ("lay-et-trill") to the market and dominated its distribution early on.

Ernst Krebs Sr., born in 1876, received a medical degree in 1903 from the San Francisco College of Physicians and Surgeons. Practicing in Nevada during the 1918 influenza pandemic, Dr. Krebs became convinced that an old Indian remedy possessed remarkable efficacy in combating the flu virus. Krebs commercialized this discovery and brought it to market as a proprietary drug named "Syrup Leptinol," which he guessed was beneficial for influenza, asthma, whooping cough, and even pulmonary tuberculosis. The label promised "miraculous results." Such an immodest claim so troubled fellow physicians that Krebs resigned from his medical societies and never rejoined. These claims also disturbed the Bureau of Chemistry agents, that were responsible for a portion of the Pure Food and Drugs Act of 1906. The Bureau had shipments of Krebs's proprietary syrup seized in Missouri, Illinois, and Oregon, claiming its label was false and fraudulent.[3]

For the next 20 to 30 years, Ernst Krebs Sr. allegedly explored in the chemistry lab a derivative of apricot seeds called amygdalin, a chemical known for a century. In 1949, Krebs's son modified his father's process by enhancing the extraction of amygdalin. Ernest Krebs Jr. then coined the name laetrile for this substance.

Earlier, Ernst Krebs Jr. had returned to California after flunking out of medical school at Hahnemann Medical College in Philadelphia. He was dismissed after having to repeat his freshman year and failing his sophomore year. He also did not have a PhD from the University of Illinois, as he asserted. His only claim to have a doctorate was an honorary doctor of science degree from the American Christian College in Tulsa, Oklahoma.[4] Ernst Krebs Jr. promoted the unorthodox theory of trophoblastic (undifferentiated cells).

He asserted that uncontrolled trophoblastic growth caused cancer, rather than the accepted paradigm that cancer is caused by invasion of abnormal cells from a body organ.[5] The theory of Krebs Jr. elaborated a mechanism by which laetrile destroyed malignant growths. Cancer cells were said to have an enzyme that freed cyanide from laetrile. Cyanide then killed cancer cells while leaving healthy cells alone. This cancer enzyme was called beta-glucosidase. In contrast, an enzyme called rhodanase protected normal body cells. Rhodanase detoxified cyanide. Conveniently, cancerous cells lack rhodanase.[6]

Theories aside, the central claim for laetrile was that it saved lives. However, only one pro-laetrile clinical study was ever published in an American medical journal. After attending a presentation on laetrile and having lunch with Krebs Jr., John Morrone MD (a private practice surgeon in New Jersey), became an enthusiast for laetrile and reported the use of laetrile in *Experimental Medicine and Surgery*, a journal no longer published.[7] Morrone concluded, "Possible regression of the malignant lesion was suggested by therapeutic results in ten cases of inoperative cancer with metastases."[8] Only three of the ten cases had biopsies reported. Morrone did not even comment on the length of survival of patients.[9] He did note pain relief (placebo effect—Chapter 13) but did not report

DOI: 10.1201/9781003324058-15

any objective parameters of the anti-cancer effect, such as size of the tumor. The trophoblastic theorists asserted that tumor size was an irrelevant parameter of treatment progress![2]

In the 1950s, the Cancer Commission of the California Medical Association sought to secure some laetrile from Krebs to permit a clinical trial. This trial would take place under the direction of the research committee and tumor board of a Los Angeles hospital. Krebs Jr. replied he was "anxious" to have clinical work commenced but foresaw difficulties. He objected to testing by physicians "ignorant of trophoblastic theory." Unless a doctor of his own choosing could direct the experiment, Krebs would send no laetrile. Such a stance occurred frequently in the next 25 years. He would demand opponents perform trials, yet when challengers offered to study laetrile, Krebs engaged in heel-dragging, refused to provide a study drug, and bickered about complying with established scientific research parameters.

The Food and Drug Administration (FDA) finally supplied its own stock of laetrile to the Cancer Commission. Controlled trials at three different cancer centers were performed for various cancers in mice. Laetrile failed to have any detectable effect. The commission also assembled as much information as possible about patients treated with laetrile—44 cases in all—and, in these cases, there was no objective evidence laetrile influenced the malignancies. The conclusion was partly based on examination of 17 cancer sufferers still alive and the autopsies of 9 of the 19 patients that had died.[10]

The commission also disputed the explanation of how laetrile purportedly functioned. The molecule-cleaving enzyme, which ostensibly released hydrogen cyanide at the site of the cancer (held by the junior Krebs to be more abundant in cancer than normal cells), was not shown to be more common. In fact, normal cells contained more of the enzyme (i.e., beta-glucosidase) than tumor tissue did. Moreover, the claim made by laetrile promoters that any dose of cyanide from laetrile was immediately detoxified to thiocyanate was disproved by the fact that cyanide is often measurable in the blood of persons who have ingested laetrile.[11] Krebs Jr. and a few laetrile physicians waved away the California Cancer Commission's report.

They said their new improved version of laetrile and better dosing levels invalidated the commission's distorted findings. In any case, they said no curative claim had ever been made. Not so. Articles quoted senior Dr. Krebs stating laetrile cured 40% of cancer patients and brought improvement to the remaining 60%.

In the 1950s, the Krebs's managed to stay under the radar of the FDA, and the use of laetrile grew modestly. This changed in 1960 when the FDA seized an interstate shipment of laetrile. In November 1961, the FDA charged Krebs Jr. with violating the law. The case did not involve laetrile, but Krebs's other major product, pangamic acid (or so-called vitamin B-15). Krebs Jr. had shipped capsules of this new drug in Florida and Oregon without prior FDA approval. He was fined $3,750 and sentenced to prison. Imprisonment was suspended when Krebs agreed to a three-year probation. One of those terms barred Krebs from manufacturing and distributing laetrile until there was an approved drug application.

PROMOTERS AND VICTIMS OF LAETRILE

Meantime, others rallied for laetrile. A writer, G. D. Kittler, penned two articles for the *American Weekly*, a Hearst publication, during March 1963. These articles presented laetrile in a most favorable light. Kittler followed these with a book entitled *Laetrile, Control for Cancer*. "The most important medical news of our time," the cover promised. The "first major breakthrough in the cancer mystery.

111

The day is near when no one needs to die from cancer. LAETRILE, the revolutionary new anti-cancer drug, will be to CANCER WHAT INSULIN IS TO DIABETES." The book presented a highly dramatic version of laetrile's discovery. Kittler considered the use of the term "cure" for cancer "inaccurate," but he added, "the idea of a cancer control on the other hand is perfectly plausible. In the minds of an increasing number of leading scientists, the best control now available is laetrile."[3]

New organizations formed to increase publicity. One group, the International Association of Cancer Victims and Friends, was founded in 1963 by a San Diego schoolteacher, Cecile Pollack Hoffman. She had turned to laetrile with despair and hope in 1959, after undergoing a radical mastectomy for breast cancer. Three years later, the spread of cancer needed further surgery. She turned to laetrile when her husband noticed a copy of Kittler's book in an airport lobby. Unavailable in the United States, Mrs. Hoffman crossed the border to Tijuana, Mexico, for laetrile injections. Persuaded that laetrile saved her life, and angry that this treatment was not legally available in the United States, Mrs. Hoffman established her international association. Through print media and group rallies, the association castigated "out of date, out-moded, the so-called 'orthodox treatment,'" and vigorously espoused what Mrs. Hoffman termed "non-toxic, beneficial therapies," especially laetrile. The organization provided cancer victims with information on how to get to Tijuana. Mrs. Hoffman died in 1969 of metastatic cancer despite the use of laetrile, but her organization plodded on.[3,12]

Others in the spirit of unorthodox treatments joined the fray. These groups lobbied for laetrile with letter-writing campaigns. One of their key themes was "freedom to use laetrile." The FDA checked its own internal judgment in 1971 by referring to an external expert opinion panel. The group of independent cancer specialists was assembled and reviewed what laetrile proponents had to offer. The conclusion of the panel was that the sum of pitiful evidence did not warrant testing in humans. Further rodent tests in recognized independent laboratories, the committee held, might be desirable. Secretary of Health, Education, and Welfare Elliott Richardson considered the conclusions of the FDA ad hoc committee valid. The secretary said, however, the National Cancer Institute would recognize grant applications for further testing by qualified independent investigators.

JOHN RICHARDSON

John Richardson began his general medical practice in the San Francisco area in 1954. After discussions with Krebs Jr., he decided to become a cancer specialist in 1971. He did not have overwhelming success as a general practitioner—his 1972 tax return revealed a taxable income of only $10,400.[3]

Becoming a cancer "expert" caused Richardson's practice to boom. He stated, "Our office soon was filled with faces we had never seen before—hopeful faces of men and women abandoned by orthodox medicine as hopeless or 'terminal cases.'" By charging $2,000 for a course of laetrile (equivalent in 2019 of about $15,000), Richardson managed to increase his income to $2.8 million between 1973 and 1976, according to his tax returns. The actual amount of money may have been even higher. In his laetrile book, he claimed he had treated 4,000 patients at an average charge of $2,500 per patient; the latter computes to $10 million.

Despite pain reduction and improved mental outlook with laetrile treatment, Richardson admitted most of his patients died. To overcome this, he massively increased the laetrile dose, added a vegetarian diet, and gave huge doses of vitamins. For this combination of diet, vitamins, and laetrile, Richardson coined the term "metabolic therapy."[3]

In 1972, Dr. Richardson was arrested at his Albany clinic (near Berkeley) and charged with prescribing laetrile in violation of the state's anti-quackery law. The dramatic arrest, filmed on television cameras, involved policemen with drawn guns and a thorough search of the premises. The physician spent a brief time in jail. A trial before a judge, finding Richardson guilty, was overturned on a technicality at appeal. Two more trials took place with hung juries. Eventually, the California Board of Medical Quality Assurance revoked Dr. Richardson's license to practice medicine in 1976 on the basis of "gross negligence and incompetence." Richardson then worked in a Mexican clinic and died of heart disease in the 1980s.

The arrest of Richardson spawned another organization led by Robert Bradford. Robert Bradford was a laboratory technician on the Stanford University staff. He formed the Committee for Freedom of Choice in Cancer Therapy (CFCCT). He gave up his Stanford job to devote full time to laetrile and the committee. In May 1976, Richardson, Bradford, and some other members of CFCCT were indicted for conspiring to smuggle laetrile. All were convicted a year later. Bradford was fined $40,000 and Richardson $20,000. It was disclosed during the trial that Bradford had paid $1.2 million for 700 shipments of laetrile, and Richardson had deposited more than $2.5 million during a 27-month period.[3]

James Harvey Young comments,

The committee and its allies focused upon freedom, making any governmental interference with a cancer sufferer's right to take any remedy available seem a violation of the constitution and the fundamental rights of man. Thus, an atmosphere of high principle infused the zealous campaign in laetrile's behalf. Laetrile's opponents, in the committee's propaganda, constituted a selfish conspiracy of those involved in orthodox cancer research and therapy, futilely cutting, burning, poisoning their victims and rejecting hopeful treatments like laetrile for fear of doing themselves out of their jobs.[2]

The campaign for laetrile then took a turn by asserting that laetrile was a vitamin and not a chemotherapy agent. Krebs Jr. apparently hoped that "vitamin" status would exempt laetrile from the safety and efficacy requirements of new drugs. However, laetrile has none of the characteristics of a vitamin. A vitamin is a substance that has been shown, when absent, to cause distinct disease manifestations, and when given back, to reverse those disease complications. The establishment of such a status depends on being shown first in the animal model and then in human beings. Nutritional scientists repeatedly pointed out that laetrile did not fulfill any criteria for a true vitamin. The vitamin ruse did not protect laetrile from action by the FDA. The manufacturers of vitamin B-17 were enjoined from distributing what the court termed both an unapproved food additive and a misbranded drug.

LEGISLATIVE SCIENCE VERSUS FREEDOM

The proponents of laetrile simultaneously turned to the legislatures for individual state laws to enable the use of laetrile. Hearings in state capitols were jammed with pro-laetrile supporters.

James Harvey Young noted in one state legislature,

Cheers greeted pro-laetrile speakers, boos and hisses their opponents. To one distinguished scientist present, "the affair appeared to be a confrontation between two cultures. One side was characterized by the voice of science—skeptical, analytical, orderly, but sometimes bluntly critical and uncompromising. The other side faced the situation with fervor, passion, conviction, revolt against logic, all emotionally expressed. They seemed to willfully reject distasteful facts."[2]

Legation and the legislative battles made laetrile an issue of national debate. Even *Sixty Minutes* (March 31, 1974) produced a segment on laetrile. By 1982, 27 states had enacted legislation to legalize laetrile.[11] Unfortunately, legislative approval gave an illusory cloak of efficacy for laetrile for the naive mind. A Harris poll showed the American public favoring legalization of laetrile by an overwhelming 30% margin.[13]

Legal battles raged. The most famous was the Rutherford case. Glen Rutherford was a 55-year-old Kansas seed salesman found to have a one-inch polyp of the colon in 1971. He was advised to have it removed after a biopsy showed it contained cancer. Fearful of surgery, he consulted Dr. Contreras in Mexico, who treated him with laetrile, vitamins, and enzymes, and cauterized (burned off) the polyp. Although cauterization almost always cures this type of cancer when it is localized in a polyp, Rutherford emerged from this experience claiming laetrile had cured him and was a necessary medicine to keep him alive. In 1975, he became the lead plaintiff in a class action suit to force the FDA to allow "terminal" cancer patients to obtain laetrile for their own use.

The case was heard before Judge Luther Bohanon in the Western Oklahoma US District Court. Bohanon was sympathetic to Rutherford's wishes. At issue were whether laetrile qualified as a grandfather drug that existed prior to the 1938 and 1962 FDA laws, and if so, whether terminally ill patients should be exempted from such regulations. The FDA reviewed the brief and determined that laetrile needed to apply for a new drug application, and thus could not be made available. Bohanon ignored the FDA and based upon the idea that denial of the drug would be an infringement of constitutionally protected rights to privacy of the plaintiffs, issued a court order in 1977 permitting individuals to import laetrile for personal use if they obtained a doctor's declaration of facts stating they were "terminally ill."[3]

Two years later, the US Supreme Court found no right to privacy in medical treatment and rejected the argument that drugs offered to "terminal" patients should be exempted from FDA regulation. The court was concerned that "if an individual suffering from a potentially fatal disease rejects conventional therapy in favor of a drug with no demonstrable curative properties, the consequences can be irreversible."[2]

However, further efforts by Rutherford and his supporters, plus defiant rulings by Bohanon, enabled the affidavit system to remain in effect until 1987, when it was finally dissolved.[3]

CHOOSING LAETRILE MEANS DELAYING CURATIVE TREATMENT

William Nolen tells a story of Mary, a 35-year-old woman, with three children, who took laetrile instead of curative orthodox therapy.[14] She presented with spotting between periods for three months. Upon examination, she had a growth on her cervix, for which biopsies proved to be a cancer. Yet, tests showed it was early and curable with radiation or surgery. She asked the usual questions about the surgery and hospitalization. Dr. Nolen answered these. She said she would call him in a few days with her decision.

When he hadn't heard in a week, he called Mary and asked what she decided. She was evasive and told Dr. Nolen she was going away for a few weeks and would be in touch when she returned. He asked her not to wait too long before deciding on therapy.

Dr. Nolen did not see her for six months. On her prior visit, Mary looked like a healthy and active young woman. When she returned, he noted a pale, thin, and sickly woman. She indicated she was now ready for radiation or surgery. Unfortunately, the tumor had spread throughout the pelvis and infiltrated the bladder. It was now untreatable. A few weeks later, Mary was dead.

What happened between her visits to Dr. Nolen? Her husband later told the story. After spending $3,000 in Mexico on a three-month treatment with laetrile, she returned home and initially looked about the same. Yet, three months after visiting Mexico, she began spotting again and losing weight. Her husband finally convinced her to see Dr. Nolen again. But it was too late.

Dr. Nolen ends his story, "Sad. Mary died a needless death, the victim of a cancer quack."[15]

TRIALS AND TOXICITY

Such was the tumult of the mass mind that a segment of sober opinion (that were unbelievers in laetrile's efficacy) concluded the fastest way to quiet public clamor would be to test laetrile in a large, prospective trial. Doing so, however, would violate the long-accepted tenet that a proponent needs to test their product first.

Officials at the National Cancer Institute also reluctantly reached the same conclusion. However, before launching a prospective trial, efforts were made to undertake a retrospective study of patients that might have benefited objectively from the use of laetrile. As reported in the *New England Journal of Medicine* in 1978, 455,000 letters were sent to physicians and health professionals attempting to find cases where patients may have responded to laetrile. No attempt was made to seek nonresponders. Of 68 cases received, only 6 were judged by an independent panel to have any possible response to laetrile. Seven were judged to have progressive cancer on laetrile. The result allowed no definite conclusions supporting the anti-cancer activity of laetrile. Despite the fact that negative responses to laetrile were not canvassed, 220 physicians sent in more than 1,000 cases that showed no response to laetrile.[16]

In the same time period, evidence was accumulating on the toxicity of laetrile. Victor Herbert points out that laetrile, or amygdalin, is 6% cyanide by weight and releases hydrogen cyanide by hydrolysis or heat in the presence of blood. The bitter almond odor, of crushed apricot kernels, is associated with release of the cyanide gas. The gas is so penetrating a poison that

> victims have died within two minutes of injection of 300 mg hydrocyanic acid in aqueous solution, an amount obtainable from two and a half ounces of some varieties of bitter almond kernels mixed with saliva, or from a sixth of an ounce of laetrile mixed with saliva in vegetables containing beta-glucosidase, a plant enzyme.[17]

The *New England Journal of Medicine* reported an 11-month-old girl that accidentally swallowed several laetrile tablets and died of cyanide poisoning.[18] Herbert recorded 15 deaths of cyanide poisoning from laetrile, along with numerous cases of toxicity with subsequent recovery. In the most pathetic case, Herbert cites a May 10, 1977, *Thousand Oaks News Chronicle* account where the author of *The Little Cyanide Cookbook*, Ms. J. Despain, fell victim to her own enthusiasm and was hospitalized comatose with acute cyanide poisoning after ingesting powder from 25 apricot kernels she had ground up, mixed with honey, and eaten (she recovered, at least physically).[17]

Under oath, two malpractice defendants in laetrile cases have refused apricot kernels offered to them with mortar and pestle to crush them.[19]

Movie star Steve McQueen attracted considerable attention when he was treated with laetrile at a Mexican clinic in 1980 under the supervision of William D. Kelley, a dentist who had been de-licensed by the State of Texas after numerous legal troubles. Although McQueen gave a glowing report when he began his treatment, he died shortly afterward.[3]

The FDA sent a warning notice in November 1977 to over one million healthcare professionals, placing them on notice that laetrile was worthless, poisonous, and often contaminated with mold. The analysis of laetrile produced in Mexico reported gives one pause—the tablets only contained 55%–87% of their stated dosage and were contaminated with debris, fungus, and bacterial products![18]

The high tide of laetrile began to recede. As mentioned previously, on June 18, 1979, a unanimous Supreme Court reversed the 10th Circuit, holding that the safety and effectiveness standards did apply to terminal patients. About the same time, the inevitable prospective clinical trial was finally started (against the advice of scientists).

Laetrile, of the type representative at the time, was used for the definitive trial. There were 178 enrollees with cancer. They were treated prospectively with laetrile, plus a "metabolic therapy" consisting of diet, enzymes, and vitamins, as was the customary practice.[20] The trial failed to detect any anti-cancer activity of laetrile. The median survival of patients was 4.8 months from the start of therapy, and in those still alive after seven months, tumor size had increased. These outcomes were the same as if no treatment had been given.

The report in the 1982, the *New England Journal of Medicine* concluded,

> no substantive benefit was observed in terms of cure, improvement, or stabilization of cancer, improvement of symptoms related to cancer, or extension of life span. The hazards of amygdalin were evidenced in several patients by symptoms of cyanide toxicity. … Amygdalin (laetrile) is a toxic drug that is not effective as a cancer treatment.[11]

The balloon popped. Laetrile had been disproved as to any possibility of effectiveness. Only a tiny core of believers remained. In a curious legal maneuver, Bradford and American Biologics (that supplied the laetrile for the National Cancer Institute [NCI] study) responded to the study with three different lawsuits against the NCI, alleging that as a result of the study, they had sustained serious financial damage due to a drastic drop in demand for laetrile! All three suits were thrown out of court.

Laetrile is still available on the Internet. Why does it still persist among us? There are many reasons. An additional reason to list is that the occasional killing from its cyanide release can easily be attributed to the underlying cancer. The coroner requests few autopsies when the patient is known to have cancer.

The reader may ask, to what ill-effect was it to finally study laetrile in proper fashion? The answer is that the laboratory and clinical research trials cost US taxpayers $375 million. This money could have easily been spent on more promising ideas in cancer treatment. Laetrile represents the first time a proponent challenged his "adversaries" to disprove his putative drug and actually goaded his adversaries into testing it!

Ernst Krebs Jr. and cohorts repeatedly accused the medical profession, FDA, and government of being an entrenched conspiracy. The truth was in fact the opposite; that is, Ernst Krebs Jr. projected his own greedy behavior upon others. At one point, Ernst Krebs Jr. was arrested with more than a million dollars of cash in his possession.

The advocates for laetrile took a dishonest approach to proof of efficacy. That is, since it was not proved or disproved, how do we know it does not help? Can we not assume it works? A quote from another era on another worthless medicine will help illustrate this idea:

> Mr. F. E. Rollins, who controls the manufacture of B. & M., believes that B. & M. (see note 21) applied to the skin and inhaled as directed, actually penetrates to the seat of the infection and kills the germs themselves. He is not a physician or a scientist. He has formed this opinion from his own personal experience on himself, by observation of others, and from what he has been told. We want to say frankly that we are not now able to prove by scientific and legally-competent evidence that this is true. Neither has it been demonstrated to our satisfaction that it is not true. Consequently, while we believe it, yet we desire clearly to be understood as making no claims or representations that B. & M. acts that way.[22]

CONCLUSION

Medical therapies should be assumed ineffective and possibly dangerous until thoroughly tested. This is not merely a supposition of a skeptic. The legitimate pharmaceutical development process has a long track record. Well-known numbers show that a promising drug has only a 1 in a 1,000 chance of surviving laboratory testing to make it to human tests; and then only a 1 in 5 chance of making it through human trials to gain FDA approval. Most drugs fail from toxicity. The organ usually harmed is the liver. So, an untested substance is more likely to harm than help.

Beyond the uncertainty gambit, why did many people believe in the unproved effectiveness of laetrile? This author suggests that in the postmodern era (proposed motto: "there are no literal truths, only voices and narratives"), many people have what is called "emotional truth." That is, something is true because their feelings indicate or wish it to be so. Certainly, the poignant picture of a suffering patient with hopeless terminal cancer arouses in us a wish that we could wave a magic wand and make the patient well.

John Leo places this tendency in perspective:

> The willingness to accept 'emotional truth,' even when it is packaged in lies, is hardly new. What's new is that those who insist on factual truth are now on the defensive, pictured as fuddy-duddies who don't understand that the self recognizes the highest truth in feelings. ... If emotional impact keeps advancing at the price of truth, we will all be in trouble.[23]

Or, as Morris Fishbein said, "The will to believe often dominates the wish to know."[24]

NOTES

1 Foundation M. *Physician's Handbook of Vitamin B17 Therapy*. Sausalito, CA: Science Press International; 1973.

2 Markle GE, Peterson JC. *Politics, Science, and Cancer: The Laetrile Phenomenon.* Boulder, CO: Westview Press; 1980, p. 1.

3 Wilson B. The rise and fall of laetrile (2004). quackwatch.org (accessed October 18, 2018).

4 A now defunct college, without a science division, never had any authority from Oklahoma to issue a doctorate degree; further, an honorary award is to be distinguished from an earned degree where actual enrollment and coursework occurs.

5 The trophoblastic hypothesis ignores the fact that most cancers show a gradual change from normal microscopic appearance to precancerous to definite cancer on the same biopsy. The source organ is thus easily identified. This process is demonstrated and learned during a course in pathology (i.e., abnormal tissues) in the second year of medical school, a course Junior never passed.

6 Later, when proof could not be found for this mechanism (and when Krebs Jr. was under court order to no longer distribute laetrile as a drug), laetrile proponents attempted to transmogrify laetrile into a vitamin (B-17).

7 Morrone JA. Chemotherapy of inoperable cancer. *Exp Med Surg* 1962;20; pp. 299–308.

8 The author reviewed this report and finds it a very poor collection of laetrile treatment anecdotes. An anecdote, in the scientific context, describes information presented in a way that cannot be quantified or compared with other studies. As one wag has said, "[T]the plural of anecdotes is not data."

9 The absolute definition of cancer requires a tissue biopsy that has been reviewed by at least two pathologists. Thus, seven of these cases may not even have had cancer.

10 Eight cases not examined to make a total of 44.

11 Moertel CG, Fleming TR, Rubin J, et al. A clinical trial of amygdalin (laetrile) in the treatment of human cancer. *New England Journal of Medicine* 1982;306; pp. 201–6.

12 Six-year survival with metastatic breast cancer is not unusual in a case such as Mrs. Hoffman's given the fact that it took four years to recur the first time. This was a slow-growing tumor, and her survival is consistent with the natural history of her tumor outcome.

13 Editorial (unsigned). Why laetrile lived so long. https://www.nytimes.com/1982/02/03/opinion/why-laetrile-lived-so-long.html

14 The reader will note the money paid in Mexico for laetrile treatment would be an equivalent to $20,000 at the time of this writing (2022).

15 Nolen, William A. *Healing: A Doctor in Search of a Miracle.* New York: Random House, 1975. pp. 32–4.

16 Ellison, Neil M, Byar David P, Newell Guy R. Special report on Laetrile: The NCI Laetrile review: Results of the National Cancer Institute's retrospective laetrile analysis. *New England Journal of Medicine* 1978;299(10); pp. 549–52.

17 Herbert, Victor. Laetrile: The cult of cyanide. Promoting poison for profit. *American Journal of Clinical Nutrition (USA)* 1979.

18 Davignon JP. Contaminated laetrile a health hazard. *New England Journal of Medicine* 1977;297; p. 1355.

19 It was an old trick of laetrile promoters to swallow the apricot pits whole in front of an audience. Of course, they would pass through the digestive tract unchanged. The exposure to cyanide comes when the seeds are ground.

20 "Metabolic" doctors were consulted.

21 B. & M. stood for Burns and McClellan, surnames of the husband and wife who advocated an old horse liniment consisting of turpentine, ammonia, eggs, and water. This 1930s doublespeak was an attempt to avoid being prosecuted for fraud under the 1906 Food and Drug Act. The latter law onerously required the government to prove the maker knowingly advocated a worthless drug. This loophole was tightened under the 1938 act. This amendment made it easier for the government to go after laetrile.

22 DeForest Lamb R, Copeland RS. *American Chamber of Horrors: The Truth about Food and Drugs*: Farrar & Rinehart; 1936, p. 65.

23 Leo J. Lying Isn't so Bad if It Makes You Feel Good. 2006. https://www. realclearpolitics.com/Commentary/com-1_22_06_JL.html (accessed October 19, 2018).

24 American Medical Association. Hygeia: American Medical Association; February 1938, p. 113.

16 Testimonials and Endorsements

We often rely on what others have experienced to guide our choices. A testimonial is a statement regarding benefits received from a treatment or product. One can hardly imagine a more effective form of publicity than a testimonial since it comes from a fellow man or woman. In the best of cases, the givers of the testimony may be sincere, or at worst con artists.

Prior to the mid-twentieth century, "proof of efficacy" in the public's mind was sufficient if one individual claimed a treatment worked for them. The advertisement worked even better if a respected community leader, such as the mayor or minister, were featured. Many patent nostrums drummed up their business by doing so.

The testimonial remains a major weapon in the arsenal of quackery. "Our experience of more than 30 years in the enforcement of the Food and Drug Act," a former FDA commissioner, W.G. Campbell, once wrote, "has demonstrated that testimonials can be obtained for practically any article labeled as a treatment for practically any disease."[1]

In the past, a claim of "miraculous" scientific breakthrough should have evoked skepticism, but often did not. Nowadays, testimonials must be much more careful in the choice of words (e.g., "cure" is out). A tanned, vigorous person endorsing the unproven herbal pill runs and leaps through a field. The implications for the product user becoming healthier are non-verbal but obvious. Celebrities are often paid for endorsements rather than common folk, though why this should improve sales is unclear.

Some examples may be helpful. The author's favorite is Figure 16.1. The Evans Vacuum Cap Company. This business existed in the early twentieth century. The device makers claimed hair could regrow by diligently applying the suction hat twice daily. The vacuum was created by means of a modified bicycle tire pump. The pump plunger was periodically pushed to maintain the vacuum. And, of course, a huge traveling case was available for the businessman.

The vacuum cap also claimed to cure dandruff and gray hair. In the days before the universal motto "to be used only as directed," several women reported using the vacuum cap to "build up their flesh and round out hollow cheeks." This led to "perceptible growth of hair" in areas where the instrument was "diligently applied" (though why women would volunteer this peculiar side effect is unclear).

The Evans Vacuum Cap Company took out advertisements in *Scientific American*. Not stated, but the implication was clear. This product was somehow scientifically based (Figure 16.2).

The author cannot dispute the separate claim of relief from constipation. The prospective client was undoubtedly reassured by the bottom line—"disposable equipment used." However, there have been reports of colonic irrigation causing perforation (a hole) in the colon, leading to at least six deaths. There have been no scientific investigations of colonic irrigation.[2]

The author grew up in Boulder, Colorado. It is home to the University of Colorado. There were an abundance of unproven treatments of every stripe, including colonic irrigation.

 DOI: 10.1201/9781003324058-16

Cosmopolitan Magazine

A Scientific Method of Growing Hair

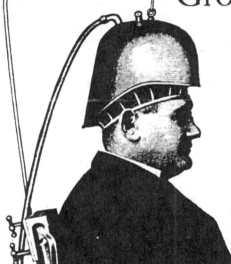

It is a known fact that the blood conveys nourishment to all parts of the body. It is likewise known that exercise makes the blood circulate, and that where the blood does *not* circulate no nourishment is supplied.

The lack of proper circulation of blood in the scalp, due mainly to congestion produced by artificial causes, results in the starvation of the hair roots, and produces falling hair and baldness. Therefore the logical and only relief from baldness is in the restoration of the scalp to its normal condition, thus enabling the blood to resume its work or nourishing the hair roots. It was work along these logical lines that produced and perfected

THE EVANS VACUUM CAP.

The Evans Vacuum Cap provides the exercise which makes the blood circulate *in the scalp.* It gently draws the rich blood to the scalp and feeds the shrunken hair roots. This causes the hair to grow. It is the simple, common-sense principles of physical culture scientifically applied to the scalp.

Easy and Pleasant to Use.

The Evans Vacuum Cap is portable and can readily be attached to any ordinary straight back chair. Three or four minutes' use each morning and evening is all that is required. It leaves a pleasant tingling sensation for a few moments after use, indicating the presence of new life in the scalp.

Method of Testing.

You can tell by a few minutes' use of the Evans Vacuum Cap whether it is possible for you to cultivate a growth of hair on your head, and we will send you the apparatus to make the experiment, *without expense on your part.* If the Evans Vacuum Cap gives the scalp a healthy glow, the normal condition of the scalp can be restored, and a three or four minutes' use of the Cap each day thereafter will, within a reasonable time, develop a natural and permanent growth of hair. If, however, the scalp remains white and lifeless after the Cap is removed, there would be no use to give the appliance a further trial. The hair cannot be made to grow in such cases.

The Bank Guarantee.

We will send you, by prepaid express, an Evans Vacuum Cap, and will allow you ample time to prove its virtue. All we ask of you is to deposit the price of the Cap in the Jefferson Bank of St. Louis, where it will remain during the trial period, subject to your own order. If you do not cultivate a sufficient growth of hair to convince you that the method is effective, simply notify the bank and they will return your deposit in full. We have no agents, and no one is authorized to sell, offer for sale or receive money for an Evans Vacuum Cap. All Caps are sold under the bank's guarantee, and all money is sent direct to Jefferson Bank.

A sixteen-page Illustrated book will be sent you free, on request.

EVANS VACUUM CAP CO.   1043 Fullerton Building, St. Louis

Figure 16.1 A vacuum cap. The cure for baldness was used twice daily for 10 minutes, according to their 16-page booklet. (Courtesy of the American Medical Association Archives, Public Domain 1905.)

THE COLONIC WORKS
Clinic for Colon Therapy

The colon is your body's sewage system. If it doesn't function properly, you don't function properly. If you have headaches, skin problems, low energy, indigestion, frequent colds or flu, hemorrhoids or infrequent bowel movements you could have a toxic condition in your colon.

Toxins from the colon can be absorbed into the blood stream and spread throughout the body perpetuating the above problems or developing into more serious problems. Colon cancer is the second most prevalent type of cancer in this country.

Colonics are a method of colon cleansing designed to remove accumulated fecal debris and toxicity. When toxins are removed, corresponding health problems are reversed. Fasting and cleansing diets are also an excellent time to consider colonics.

Benefits From Colon Therapy Include Relief and Elimination From the Following:

Gas	Tension
Constipation	Depression
Headaches	Abdominal Distension
Food Cravings	Restlessness
Skin Problems	Dark CirclesUnder Eyes
Not feeling well	Sallow Complexion

For information and appointments contact:
Jane Doe, 720-555-1234
Disposable Equipment Used (!?)

Figure 16.2   Example of an advertisement for colonic irrigation. (Author composed this generic flier.)

Strange to say, university towns are hotbeds of quackery. Too often the professor thinks that because he knows a lot about mathematics or Greek, he automatically knows a lot about medicine.[3]

More recently, a Hollywood actress hypes a colon cleanse regimen in—*Is Gwyneth Paltrow Wrong About Everything?—How the Famous Sell Us Elixirs of Health, Beauty and Happiness*. The technique uses a rectal enema, and the injected liquid is coffee. (We will not illustrate this.) Despite the packets costing $425, and no scientific evidence, demand for this product remains strong.[4]

Old ideas die hard. The Egyptians 4,000 years ago felt that stool contents were the source of all disease.

THE FOUR CHALLENGES OF A TESTIMONIAL

When considering the veracity of a testimonial, there are four considerations. Does the person actually exist? If so, do they have the alleged disease? Is the promotor of the treatment qualified? Finally, has this treatment been tested with proven results?

IS THE TESTIFIER REAL?

The American Medical Association's (AMA) Department of Investigation existed from 1912 to 1975. In a time before government agencies were policing health fraud, the AMA performed this task. Their *Historical Health Fraud and Alternative Collection* exposes scores of bogus people that gave a testimonial.[5]

It would be humorous, if not so serious, when endorsements are given for a product, only to find out the patient has died of the disease shortly thereafter. Even worse are the testimonials where the patient died before the date of the advertisement (see following). Upon follow-up, many people used for testimonials were unaware they were being used for an advertising campaign.

THE DUTCH TAKE HOLLAND

Testimonials can also fall into "cases of the Dutch taking over Holland!"[6] That is, the patients never had tuberculosis (or whatever disease).[7] This assertion cannot be carried too far. Patients often equate symptoms with self-diagnosed disease. For example, spitting up blood must mean cancer of the tongue, whereas there are scores of possible diagnoses. Or the physician reports a shadow on a radiological exam and recommends a follow-up test. The patient assumes the doctor is being kind by not coming straight out with the cancer diagnosis. The patient then starts taking vitamin "X." The follow-up test shows no shadow. The patient credits vitamin X for curing his or her cancer. As Young puts it, "To the quack and his most susceptible victims, all coughs are consumption, all lumps, cancer, and all backaches, kidney disease."[8]

In Healing: A Doctor in Search of a Miracle, William Nolan, a Catholic surgeon, chronicled his honest search for a verifiable case of miraculous healing. The 15 cases submitted to him by patients in response to canvassing were reviewed. In almost every case, it was difficult for Dr. Nolan to determine whether the patient actually had the disease claimed to have been cured. In the one case with biopsy-proven prostate cancer, the patient, in addition to his religious efforts, had also received standard medical therapy; the two sources of relief confound the ability to credit the source of recovery.[9,10]

One New York newspaper even published a statement for Sargon, an elixir with an alcohol content of 18%. The paper ran this testimonial as a news article on June 25, 1930. The headline ran "Labor Official Praises Sargon for New Health." James Kimber, of 314 Winton Road, Rochester, reported how he had gained 18 pounds in 6 weeks. He had been having trouble sleeping, nausea, and constipation. He was quoted as saying,

> I felt myself gaining ground right from the first few doses of Sargon: as I "snapped out" of my troubles I gradually got my weight back and the feeling of strength and energy that's come with it is impossible to describe.

Apparently, the news department at the paper did not communicate well with the obituary section. Five days earlier, on June 20, 1930, James Kimber's obituary was run in the same newspaper. The article related that James Kimber, former alderman and prominent Mason, died suddenly the day before at his home, 314 Winton Road, aged 62 years. He had not looked well for several months but had been coming to work.[11]

Another facet of the Dutch taking Holland is outright fraud. The old dictum still stands, "If you want a really good testimonial, write it yourself."[12]

> Between the steel exterior and porcelain interior of this [drinking] mug lies a material that magnetizes hot or cold liquids. Why? Because magnetizing water, the basis of any liquid, creates space between its molecules, adding alkalinity to water that has become acidic. Alkaline water is more readily absorbed by the body.[13]

This is utter nonsense. Only iron has magnetic properties. Creating space between molecules cannot occur. It will not make water more alkaline. The body does not absorb alkaline water more readily.[13]

Unqualified and Misunderstood Practitioners

Advocates with bogus credentials give bad treatment. John Brinkley and the Krebs father-son duo are prime examples. The credentials of these latter men were falsified. Other sincere proponents of laetrile, for example, failed to notice the lack of trained expertise in these men. When challenged, the diversionary tactic of quacks is the "Galileo ploy"; meaning we "are misunderstood because our ideas are ahead of time," implying that any critic is a dinosaur.

> Physicians pooh-poohed such pretensions, especially on the part of market-ers who lacked even a scintilla of scientific nature. … "Who would employ a blacksmith to repair a watch, a barber to shoe a horse, a ship-carpenter to make bonnets, or a milliner to build a church?"[14]

Quacks often set a smokescreen of yelling corruption toward big pharma while simultaneously counting their huge stacks of money. The reader will recall Krebs Jr. of laetrile fame being arrested with the more than $1 million in cash.

The author went to medical school at Washington University in St. Louis, where there were legendary stories of the surgeon "50 Cent Smith." His moniker derived from his charge of 50 cents per operation during the 1920s and 1930s. Fifty Cent Smith would make a sham skin incision over the afflicted organ site, such as the left lower quadrant of the abdomen for the appendix; sew it up; and claim he had removed the appendix and saved the patient's life from appendicitis. His patients adored him.

The County Medical Society attempted for years to get 50 Cent Smith barred from practice, but they could never find a dissatisfied patient willing to testify against the sham surgeon. Still, his patients trickled into St. Louis City Hospital during later decades. Sometimes, they required abdominal operations for other reasons. Imagine the astonishment of a surgeon at laparotomy when the preoperative history of the patient noted the patient had his appendix removed 30 years earlier and then to discover his appendix was still present! This happened many times.

Yet, on one occasion, 50 Cent Smith was stuck having to produce a tangible result by performing a cesarean section. This created the obvious need to deliver a baby. He did so. But then he was perplexed about what to do with the soccer ball–sized uterus (apparently not being aware it will rapidly shrink). His next decision was clear from follow-up surgery 40 years later. A narrow band of scarred uterus stretched from the xiphoid process (inferior point of the sternum or chest bone) some 40 centimeters (16 inches) to its origin in the pelvis. This compares to the uterus's usual length of 6–7 centimeters or 2–3 inches. Smith must have decided the uterus needed to be sewn to the xiphoid process for support!

Snake Oil Medicine

"Snake oil medicine" means the proposed medicine does not contain an active ingredient. In the past, it also included patent medicines with a high amount of alcohol content. Most people do not understand that current over-the-counter "alternative medicines" or those sold as "complementary medicines" are not regulated or tested. The ingredients listed on the container may or may not be in the container—they are subject only to the scruples of the manufacturer. When ginseng products were analyzed, for example, the amount of the active ingredient in each pill varied by as much as tenfold among brands labeled as containing the same amount. Some brands contained none at all.[15] The FDA can only intervene after the fact when reports of toxicity or body counts rise. An editorial in the *New England Journal of Medicine* opined,

> What most sets alternative medicine apart, in our view, is that it has not been scientifically tested, and its advocates largely deny the need for such testing. … [They] believe the scientific method is simply not applicable to their remedies. They rely instead on anecdotes and theories.[15]

The reason testing is not done is that it costs time and money. In the short term, it is simply the outlay of money to run controlled trials. Currently, the cost of entering patients into a randomized controlled trial is more than a thousand dollars apiece. Two hundred and fifty patients would mean a quarter of a million dollars.

For example, a colleague of the author wished to study an herbal medicine purported to help liver disease in humans. He needed to obtain a standard preparation of the herb and a look-alike placebo for study. When he finally tracked down the owner of the company, the owner replied, "Why should I study a medication when I already make two million dollars a year from it? It is possible the study may prove negative and I will lose my income."

Indeed. Let the suckers pay.

That a treatment is "natural" in origin adds no value. The apricot pit substance, laetrile, can release cyanide. There may be no more effective human poison than cyanide. Other examples of natural yet harmful substances would be arsenic or hemlock.

Second, mentioning that a therapy is ancient is also no recommendation. With only a few exceptions, therapies from the distant past are unproven. Moreover, most untested medicines whose candidacy appears promising fail testing in human trials.

CASE REPORTS VERSUS ANECDOTES

Physicians refer to individual outcomes as case reports. Case reports can answer unique clinical questions directly, report novel toxicities, or report rare diseases. Anecdotes do not allow comparison. That is, they lack enough data for comparison. On the other hand, a case report provides enough scientific information to compare to other cases. The author has published the following case reports.[16]

Case One: Can I Take My Psychiatric Medicine and Breastfeed My Child?

Ms. A, a 36-year-old mother of one child, had been taking amitriptyline for ten years to control her depression. Her usual dose, 150 mg/day, was decreased to 100 mg/day when her second pregnancy was discovered. Ms. A had suffered severe postpartum depression (i.e., suicidal) after the birth of her first child. Because she wanted to breastfeed her second child, she asked if she should continue taking amitriptyline. The author did not know the answer but review of the medical literature was of no help. With consent, the author obtained for the laboratory timed samples of mother's blood, breast milk, and baby's blood. Research testing showed the same levels in the mother's blood and breast milk (1/10,000th of the ingested dose), but amitriptyline was undetectable in the baby's serum. Thus, Ms. A was advised breastfeeding was safe.[17]

Comment: Given the life-threatening nature of her postpartum depression and the benefits of breastfeeding, the question was worthy of investigating. This resulted in exact clinical advice. Amitriptyline is still widely used for many purposes. The unusual feature of this investigation was the determination of the drug in breast milk, an examination rarely performed, and much of the article defended the milk assay's methodology. The decisive factor was that any amount added to breast milk could be detected by the assay.[17] The value of this modest study has persisted. Sixty-seven scientific articles have cited it in the last 40 years, and as recent as 2016.[18]

Case Two: High on Chromic Acid?

Metallic chromium is used to plate car bumpers or in stainless steel products. Acute chromium ingestion causes a clinical syndrome of gastroenteritis, toxic hepatitis, and renal failure. It has been fatal in 6 of 13 cases reported in the literature of patients treated with peritoneal dialysis or hemodialysis. Before the advent of dialysis, this syndrome was uniformly fatal. This report provided the first description of an intravenous injection of chromic acid causing acute renal failure.

A 31-year-old male prisoner injected an unknown amount of an industrial cleaning compound composed of 60% chromic acid and 40% potassium fluozirconate. He was a drug addict who thought he could get "high on the acid!" He had a history of intravenous drug abuse of heroin, cocaine, and "anything else I can get my hands on." When asked later why this substance was injected, he replied, "I thought acid was acid." For the next three days, he suffered nausea, vomiting, dark red urine, and loose reddish stools. Seven days after injection, he reported for medical care with the chief complaint of depression and was admitted to the prison psychiatric service. A medical consultation revealed evidence for acute renal failure. He was sent to a dialysis center in a local hospital for 15 days. Eight days after the injection, his urine chromium level was 3,640 mcg/mL (expected 0–10 mcg/mL).[19] During his hospital stay, he developed a pulmonary embolism. After three months, he made a complete recovery.[20]

Comment: This intravenous injection of the heavy metal chromium would never be allowed in human experimentation. Thus, the author felt a responsibility to publish it, as it would fill out the spectrum of poisonings from chromium. It is hoped the patient's proclivity to inject unknown acids has ceased.

Case Three: A New Type of Hepatitis Approaches the United States

The author reported a suspected case of hepatitis E to the Centers for Disease Control (CDC) in March 1991. Hepatitis E, a recently discovered virus, was causing outbreaks of jaundice in the Soviet Union, Africa, and near Mexico City, but not in the United States. A 38-year-old woman from Denver, Colorado, traveled 30 miles south of Tijuana to Rosarito Beach, Mexico, for one day. She ingested four alcoholic margaritas with crushed ice. The ice was the source of infection. She soon returned to Denver, and three weeks later became ill and developed jaundice. Tests were sent to the CDC and returned positive for hepatitis E. Her symptoms and liver tests resolved 30 days later.[21]

Comment: Hepatitis E is an enteric infection (i.e., caught by oral ingestion) of the liver that causes significant illness for two to three weeks but resolves. The only people that die from it are women who catch the infection during pregnancy. This is an example of a sentinel report, which alerts physicians of an infection or disease that is occurring in or near the area they practice. The idea is that one cannot recognize a problem if there is no awareness of the possible diagnosis.[22]

UNLIKELY SURVIVORS

Diseases in which there is no effective treatment are of great interest when a favorable outcome occurs. This author keeps waiting for a poor soul to have biopsy-proven metastatic carcinoma of the pancreas and then claim they are a five-year survivor after taking compound "X." The natural history of metastatic pancreatic cancer is to be dead in one to three years, with or without treatment. It would be remarkable for such a patient to survive five years. Such a claim, if verified, should prompt further consideration.

The first patient treated with penicillin is a case in point. In Oxford, England, Dr. Charles Fletcher treated Albert Alexander, a 43-year-old policeman, on February 12, 1941. Alexander had been injured in a bombing raid. His wounds became infected and complicated by septicemia (i.e., seeding of the infection into the bloodstream). His prognosis was grave. He was expected to die within days.

Fletcher injected Alexander regularly with penicillin over four days. Even though the doses were tiny by today's standard, Alexander started getting better: his fever dropped; his appetite returned; the infected wound began to heal. Because of a limited supply, the team went as far as extracting the precious penicillin from his urine and reinjecting it. Unfortunately, supplies ran out before his cure was complete. He relapsed at the beginning of March and died a month later. Soon though, four more seriously ill patients recovered with penicillin.[23] When dramatic recovery occurs in a few cases certain to die, further investigation is warranted.

CONCLUSION

The testifier to a treatment may be bogus, dead, or an unwitting subject. The "doctor" may have dubious credentials. The treatment is often untested, toxic, or phony. If the claimed pill has not been examined scientifically, it means the user is being experimented on. When the quack says, "How do you know this doesn't help?" the response should be, "How do you know it does not harm?"[24] If the reader thinks human nature has evolved to a higher state of ethics or morals, then they are naive. Snake oil salesmen will always be around to drain our bank accounts, if not damage our health.

On the other hand, case reports by qualified observers can provide valuable information about toxicity. If dramatic positive treatment effects occur, more testing is needed before recommendations can be made.

NOTES

1 Young JH. *American Health Quackery: Collected Essays of James Harvey Young*. Princeton University Press; 2014, p. 4.

2 Barrett S. Gastrointestinal quackery: Colonics, laxatives, and more. 2010. https://www.quackwatch.org/01QuackeryRelatedTopics/gastro.html (accessed October 30, 2018).

3 Alvarez W. The appeal of quackery to the nervous invalid. *Minnesota Medicine* 1933:16; p. 87.

4 Caulfield T. *Is Gwyneth Paltrow Wrong about Everything? When Celebrity Culture and Science Clash*. Toronto, Canada: Penguin Canada; 2015.

5 *Historical Health Fraud and Alternative Collection*. Chicago, IL: American Medical Association Archives.

6 Apologies to the Dutch.

7 DeForest Lamb R, Copeland RS. *American Chamber of Horrors: The Truth about Food and Drugs*. New York: Farrar & Rinehart; 1936, p. 65.

8 Young JH. *The Medical Messiahs*. Princeton, NJ: Princeton University Press; 1967, p. 425.

9 Of course in severe illness both medical treatment and religious effort can be pursued. Medical treatment should never be ignored. The author's position is fully explained in "John Wesley and Science" in—*Wesleyans Help Women's Suffrage* Teddy Bader. Amazon.com, 2018.

10 Nolen WA. *Healing: A Doctor in Search of a Miracle*. New York: Random House; 1975, p.93.

11 Cramp AJ. *Nostrums and Quackery and Pseudo Medicine*. Chicago: American Medical Association; 3; 1936, p. 201.

12 Jameson E. *The Natural History of Quackery*. London: Michael Joseph Publishing; 1961, p. 160.

13 Barrett S. Questionable ads for magnets. https://quackwatch.org/related/PhonyAds/magnetad/; September 18, 1989 (accessed May 9, 2022).

14 Young, 2014, p. 38.

15 Angell M, Kassirer J. Alternative medicine—The risks of untested and unregulated remedies. *New England Journal of Medicine* 1998;339; pp. 839–41.

16 Presented in summary fashion. For full report see reference number.

17 Bader T, Newman K. Amitriptyline in human breast milk and the nursing infant's serum. *American Journal of Psychiatry* 1980;137; pp. 855–6.

18 Google Scholar searched March 25, 2019.

19 His kidneys positively "glowed" on the radiographs.

20 Bader TF. Acute renal failure after chromic acid injection. *Western Journal of Medicine* 1986;144; pp. 608–9.

21 Bader TF, Krawczynski K, Polish LB, Favorov MO. Hepatitis E in a United States traveler to Mexico. *New England Journal of Medicine* 1991;325; p. 1659.

22 After publication in the *New England Journal of Medicine*, the author was awakened one night by a call from a man with a slight Mexican accent who identified himself as the district attorney of Tijuana (Mexico). He asked which hotel in Rosarito Beach the woman had visited. When I refused to tell him, he asked follow-up questions as one might expect from a

prosecuting attorney. I became concerned that some type of extreme action might be taken against the hotel (i.e., blow up the building). Finally, I told him he had to contact the CDC for further details. He hung up.

23 Barrett M. Penicillin's first patient: Uncovering the truth behind the first man treated with the world's first antibiotic. https://mosaicscience.com/story/penicillin-first-patient-history-albert-alexander-AMR-DRI/ (accessed November 12, 2018).

24 Barrett S, Jarvis WT. *Health Robbers*. Dallas, TX: Prometheus Books; 1993, p. 24.

17 Controlled Trials and Hidden Harm

Sherlock Holmes related,

> While the individual man is an insoluble puzzle, in the aggregate, he becomes a mathematical certainty. You can, for example, never foretell what any man will do, but you can say with precision what an average number will be up to. Individuals vary, but percentages remain constant. So says the statistician.[1]

Natural history is the expected course of a disease without intervention. The understanding of natural history involves following a group of people with that disease over many years. The natural history must be well understood to ensure that the control group is not under- or overperforming. The control group used during the study should perform in a manner similar to that reported in the scientific literature. For example, we know that 40% of people that present with a stomach ulcer will heal their ulcer on their own in eight weeks without any medication. Sixty percent will not heal. This is good for a physician to know, but it does not help predict if a particular individual will heal spontaneously.

The need to compare the outcome of treatments between an untreated group and a group of people that receive the test medication comprises the idea of a "controlled" trial. This term is the most important word in the phrase "randomized, double-blind, placebo-controlled trial" (RCT). Surprisingly, there are only a few sources on the history of the RCT, and these contain limited discussions. Why this lack exists is not evident to the author. Writings about the surefire way of combating disease should be so common that we tire of it.

In any case, the earliest understanding of this process revolves around the controlled trial. In its simplest form, an evaluator takes two groups and gives one group the interventional treatment. The second group is a control group and has not received any intervention. The control group is observed in the same manner as the test group. At the end of a predetermined time, the two groups are evaluated for clearly defined and reliable responses. Obvious differences that are either favorable or unfavorable, then support or negate the use of the tested treatment.

The variations of this basic approach are legion. Few trials nowadays have untreated controls. Instead, the control group may be assigned the standard method of treatment for the condition. In the latter case, the test group may be a new treatment. Or the control group may receive a different dose of the medicine or a placebo (Chapter 13). A control group helps account for individual variation, natural history of disease, and possible adverse effects of the proposed treatment. Whether the standard treatment for the condition is given to the control group depends on the amount of scientific evidence for that treatment. If there is poor evidence for the standard of therapy, then a placebo is certainly a valid choice.

One can never account for what is happening in an individual given a treatment. The changes observed may have occurred even if the treatment had not been done. For example, physicians are taught that given a hundred persons with a well-defined disease at a particular stage, 30 will recover, 40 will have progressive injury, and 30 will die within a year. At the same time, when a physician confronts an individual, he or she must humbly admit they cannot give any precise information other than the large group outcome. Nevertheless, follow-up of the single individual, for even a brief period, will begin to make the course clearer.

DOI: 10.1201/9781003324058-17

DANIEL IN THE KING'S COURT

Historical examples help illustrate these ideas.

The earliest record of a controlled trial is the Hebrew story in the Book of Daniel. In this story, "young men without any physical defect, handsome, showing aptitude for every kind of learning, well informed, quick to understand, and qualified to serve in the king's palace [i.e., the King of Babylon, Nebuchadnezzar]" were to be trained for three years to enter the king's service. The king assigned them a portion of royal food and wine from his table for their rations. For religious reasons, Daniel and his three friends from Judah asked the king's supervisor to be exempted from this diet.

The official replied, "I am afraid of my Lord the King, who has assigned your food and drink. Why should he see you looking worse than the other young men your age? The King would have my head because of you." Instead, Daniel proposed a diet limited to vegetables and water. He begged the supervisor to wait 10 days. Then he could compare the [test] group of four men to the remaining [control] group consuming the royal food and wine. Then "treat [judge] your servants in accordance with what you see."

After ten days, the foursome "looked healthier and better nourished than any of the young men who ate the royal food." Daniel and his friends won their exemption from the king's menu.

Interestingly, the story from Daniel specifies seven defining characteristics of the test participants. These are now called inclusion and exclusion criteria. These distinctive qualities are necessary to define the groups undergoing testing. In this case, an exclusion would have been any young man with a "defect" (whatever that meant). The six inclusion criteria were to be a well-informed, handsome, young man from Judah, who showed an aptitude for learning and was quick to understand. Finally, the young man under consideration had to be "qualified to serve in the king's palace." The reader may be amused at the ambiguity of the foregoing criteria, but the examples illustrate that criteria clear to one investigator can appear imprecise to another.

VITAMIN C AND SCURVY

James Lind's test of lemons for treatment of scurvy in British sailors onboard a ship during 1747 was a landmark study. Scurvy is a debilitating disease characterized by swelling and bleeding of the gums in the mouth, extensive bleeding spots on the skin, and severe fatigue. Bed rest was inevitable. As time went on, the afflicted sailor would develop acute heart failure and die unless the ship reached port. The devastation to the British navy during the years between 1500 and 1800 was enormous. Although exact statistics are not available on naval mortality, most observers at the time, and historians now, think that scurvy caused more sailor deaths than naval battles, shipwreck, and all other diseases combined![2]

Two hundred years earlier, scurvy was first noticed in the initial long-term sea voyages of the Spanish. Afflicted men got better when their ships docked, so it was believed the disease took place on extended voyages because men were land creatures and not sea creatures; their prolonged absence from land was the problem.

As a ship's surgeon, James Lind was shaken by the return to England, in 1744, of an around-the-world voyage undertaken by Captain Anson. Three-quarters of the crew died, mostly due to scurvy.[3]

Lind describes his own controlled trial,

On the 20th of May 1747, I saw twelve patients with scurvy on board the *HMS Salisbury* at sea. Their cases were as similar as I could have them.

They all had putrid and bloody gums, with hemorrhagic spots all over; their weakness was so great they were confined to their beds. They lay together in one place, being a proper apartment for the sick in the fore-hold; and had one diet in common to all, namely, water gruel sweetened with sugar in the morning; fresh mutton broth for dinner; at other times puddings, boiled biscuit with sugar etc.; and for supper barley, raisins, rice and currants, and wine. [The experiment being] that two men were ordered each a quart of cider a day. Two others took 25 drops of elixir vitriol[4] three times a day. Two others took two spoonfuls of vinegar three times a day. Two of the patients were put under a course of sea water. Of this they drank half a pint every day. Two others ate two oranges and one lemon every day. However, the ship supplies only allowed the fruit for six days before running out. The two remaining patients took the bigness [sic] of a nutmeg three times a day.[5] The consequence was that the most sudden and visible good effects were perceived from the use of the oranges and lemons; one of those who had taken them being at the end of six days fit for duty. The spots were not indeed at that time quite off his body, nor his gums sound; but without any other medicine, other than a gargle for his mouth, he became quite healthy before we came into Plymouth, which was on the 16th of June. The other man taking oranges was the best recovered and was appointed nurse to the other sick men.[6]

All six experimental arms included treatments deemed by others, in uncontrolled observations, helpful in the treatment of scurvy. Despite placing only two sailors in each group, the results were clear. The effect of the citrus fruit was dramatic, and the effect of the other treatments was nil. This shows that many patients need not be tested if the favorable effect is dramatic. Lind also standardized the condition of the trial well. They were kept in the same part of the ship and all given the same diet.

One strength of the controlled trial is that the investigator's theory need not be right in order to find an efficacious treatment. Modern withdrawal experiments have shown that scurvy is a disease of vitamin C deficiency. As others of his age, Lind believed scurvy was due to the miasmatic atmosphere of extreme humidity on shipboard, which caused an inability to respond with normal perspiration. He reasoned the moist air blocked sweat glands from exuding a disease causing an internal toxin. To counter this, lemon juice acted as a detergent that divided the toxic particles so they could slip through the constricted sweating pores in the skin.[7]

Despite his report to the British Admiralty, it took 48 years (until 1795) for the tradition-bound service to start using lemons. This delay was partly due to the lack of understanding of what constituted proof of efficacy. Nevertheless, the British navy was well ahead of other navies by instituting lemons or limes for their sailors. In a single stroke—by prescribing limes—England doubled the size of its naval manpower. The limes provided enough able manpower for the British navy to defeat the scurvy-ridden fleet of Napoleon at the momentous battle of Trafalgar in 1805.

While Lind performed his testing in obscurity, the reader may recall the next trial done by Louis Pasteur in Chapter 9, where 25 sheep were given the anthrax vaccine and 25 sheep were used as controls. All were inoculated with anthrax. The trial was done in the limelight of the media. After 26 days, all the unvaccinated sheep given anthrax died. Whereas none of the vaccine group challenged with anthrax died.

The scurvy and anthrax trials demonstrate that when treatment effects are large, small numbers are convincing.

PERCENTAGES OR FREQUENCIES?

It is surprising how many people struggle with percentages. A hidden video of a dress for sale in a boutique shop on a Los Angeles sidewalk was made. To make it simple, the dress was priced at $100. Passersby were told the dress on sale was 50% off. For what would it actually sell? To supply motivation, the quizzed person was told he or she could have either the dress or the cash amount for the correct answer. The first 10 adult respondents could not guess the right price. Dollar amounts of $30, $40, or more were volunteered. The 11th man guessed the correct amount of $50 and won the prize. This incident reinforces another poll that eight out of ten adult Americans have difficulty calculating a percentage.

Then, there is the confusion about a probability statement:

> This happens even with such familiar statements as "there is a 30 percent chance it will rain tomorrow." Some think it will rain 30 percent of the time, others that it will rain in 30% of the area, and a third group believes it will rain on 30% of the days like tomorrow. These three interpretations are about equally frequent. What weather forecasters have in mind is the last interpretation. However, people should not be blamed for different interpretations; the statement "there is a 30 percent chance it will rain tomorrow" is ambiguous.[8]

The results are better apprehended as a frequency, rather than a percentage. That is, when people are told there is a one in three chance of it raining tomorrow, a far greater percentage concludes the intended probability that it will rain on one out of three days like tomorrow.

HEAD COLDS

Similarly, controlled trials help us avoid erroneous conclusions based on incorrect science. A hundred different strains of viruses cause head colds. Members of the rhinovirus genus are most common. However, in the 1930s, little was known about viruses and how they caused disease. In one of the very earliest RCTs, reported in 1938, Dr. Diehl and a group from Minneapolis gave a "cold vaccine" to 272 college students who believed themselves predisposed to head colds. The control group with 276 students was given an injection of sodium chloride. The composition of the cold vaccine was not of a nature that we would now think had anything to do with an upper respiratory infection. The vaccine was composed of killed bacteria of four species. There were no viral components. Did the injection of four killed bacteria species work as a vaccine (Table 17.1)?

Table 17.1 Results of a Trial of Killed Bacteria Vaccine versus Controls

Cold Vaccine Trial in College Students	Vaccine	Control
Volunteers in each group	272	276
Average number of colds per person		
Previous year	5.9	5.6
Current year	1.6	2.1
Reduction per 100 subjects	73	63

Note: Without a control group, it appears that the vaccine group, with a 73% reduction, had significant protection from head colds until we see the group that received placebo injections lowered theirs by 63%.

133

The differences between groups were inconsequential. But what if there had been no control group? The 73% reduction in the vaccine group would have been impressive.[9]

CONTROLS CAN REVEAL TOXICITY

Another reason for having a control group is to observe unsuspected side effects. One example was a controlled trial of using interferon and ribavirin in patients with chronic renal failure for treatment of hepatitis C. Hepatitis C patients, without kidney problems, given interferon and ribavirin usually clear the virus in 50%, or 1 in 2 subjects. However, the treatment appeared ineffective to most clinicians when given to patients with chronic renal failure. Still, there was a minority of clinicians who advocated that hepatitis C patients with chronic renal failure should be treated. These hepatitis C patients, it was alleged, should experience a cure rate equal to those without kidney problems. There was a handful of published case reports to support the practice in kidney patients.

The National Institutes of Health organized a RCT study using interferon alone in one arm compared to interferon and ribavirin in a second arm. The issue at stake was that the kidneys excreted ribavirin, and this was a principal reason it was not used for fear of accumulation in the bloodstream of patients with advanced kidney disease. Despite starting with low doses of ribavirin and increasing the dose gradually, the trial was stopped after 13 patients were enrolled. One patient in the interferon and ribavirin arm had a grand mal seizure and died. The review panel felt the death was due to the accumulation of ribavirin in the bloodstream, resulting in a fatal convulsion. While the primary reason the trial was stopped was the one death from ribavirin, the other judgment was that only one of the other 12 patients had any antiviral (i.e., lowered level of hepatitis C virus) response.

Patients with advanced kidney disease have a poor prognosis and die from many causes. Had this individual been treated outside a controlled trial, the death could have easily been attributed to a complication of the kidney disease itself, not the ribavirin. Clinicians often find another reason for death in an individual with advanced organ disease, rather than the therapy itself. This is not dishonesty. This is the complexity of attempting to tease out what the advanced disease is doing versus the effect of treatment. Since clinicians are altruistic, it is always easier to find another cause. If the injury is not fatal, the therapy can be discontinued to determine if the damaging effect is reversible. When the patient dies, a replay is not possible.

A major problem in the scientific medical literature is that only positive treatment effects are published. Editors are not interested in publishing interventional studies that did not work. Subscribers are not interested in reading failed trials.

Returning to our example, there are a few anecdotal reports of patients with advanced kidney disease that were cured of their hepatitis C infection when given interferon and ribavirin. However, it is likely that this effort was achieved through a fog of patients who failed treatment or died. The failures would not be submitted for publication, while the rare success would be.

GOLD FOR TUBERCULOSIS

In the 1920s, as many as one in five people were actively infected with tuberculosis. Moreover, there was no proven benefit of any medicine. In this setting, the introduction of a medicine claiming to cure tuberculosis grabbed headlines. Gold thiosulfate, popularly named Sanocrysin, contained 37% gold. Gold-plated hopes for healing fueled a lust for the magical compound.

Sanocrysin was first developed by Holger Mollgäard, a professor at the Royal College in Copenhagen. In 1924, his experiments were published in a volume titled *The Chemotherapy of Tuberculosis: Experimental Foundation and Preliminary Clinical Results*. In it, he reported Sanocrysin to be a powerful and dangerous drug. Among other serious problems, it caused a reaction he called "Sanocrysin shock," in which some animals rapidly developed heart and lung failure before dying. Mollgäard theorized this was from the release of tubercle toxins when so many bacilli were killed quickly. He supposed this reaction could be reduced with the use of tuberculin serum prepared from animals. When Sanocrysin and tuberculin serum were combined, Mollgäard claimed Sanocrysin had a significant curative effect.[10]

Not surprisingly, uncontrolled trials in humans produced enthusiastic reports. The late 1920s produced many trials of Sanocrysin, described as "controlled" trials, but with vague end points and poor follow-up, they were no better than anecdotes. It wasn't until 1940 that the report of Martini and Rosen specified 11 criteria that would bring the criteria for a controlled trial for TB into modern equivalence.[11]

An exception to the general weak methodology in controlled TB trials was a trial in Detroit by James Burns, Amberson, and colleagues reported in 1931. Contemporaries, as well as later historians, recognized this trial for its scientific rigor.[12] In 1926, Amberson, with the Detroit Municipal Tuberculosis Sanatorium, asked for volunteers afflicted with pulmonary tuberculosis. Amberson chose 24 patients. On the basis of clinical, laboratory, and X-ray findings, two groups were divided into two comparable groups of 12 each. Then, by a flip of a coin, one group became identified as group I (recipients of Sanocrysin, sodium-gold-thiosulfate) and the other as group II (control). Sanocrysin was given by injection; control patients received injections of distilled water.[12]

Participants were not told whether they were being treated with the active drug. This is what is meant by blinding in a trial. It does not mean the patients cannot see, it is that they do not know if they are getting the active treatment or being used as a control. The Sanocrysin trial may represent the first time the precept of single blindness was used in a clinical trial.

Sanocrysin neither helped nor harmed the tuberculosis infection compared to the control group. During the trial, all patients in the Sanocrysin group suffered temporary renal injury, and one ended up with permanent kidney damage. One patient in the Sanocrysin arm died of liver failure. This was judged a toxic drug reaction. Amberson called it "gold poisoning." Again, if the fatal liver case or kidney damage had been under individual treatment, the problems could have been fobbed off as caused by tuberculosis or happenstance.[12]

Others had noted the common occurrence of kidney damage when using Sanocrysin. Mollgäard's idea that an injection of Sanocrysin caused shock because it rapidly killed so many TB bacilli was falling from favor. Besides, even if the allegation were true, the patient often died along with the bacilli. A Pyrrhic victory. The use of gold salts for the treatment of TB began declining in the 1930s to disappear by 1940. This was due in large measure to another treatment option, artificial pneumothorax, appearing more beneficial and less hazardous than gold therapy. Yes, the reader read the last line correctly. Introducing considerable amounts of air into the chest cavity, causing the collapse (and nonfunction or partial function) of one lung, was safer than gold treatment. The idea was to rest the lung and decrease oxygen delivery to the TB bacillus. The surgical intervention seemed to help. However, there have never been any prospective controlled trials of pneumothorax for TB.

ARE THE COMPARED GROUPS SIMILAR?

The absolute basis for a valid comparison in the test and control groups is that these two groups are equivalent. Or, in the vernacular, we need to compare apples with apples, not apples and oranges. In the case of medical investigation, the two groups must represent the same disease. There is no such thing as groups being perfectly identical, but one must not allow a major force to impact one and not the other. As mentioned earlier, inclusion and exclusion criteria are important to ensure that we compare similar groups. Doctors may have different criteria for diagnosing a particular disease. Therefore, the list of inclusion and exclusion criteria helps ensure that the groups are reasonably similar.

Bias in selection of patients is always a hazard. Despite inclusion criteria, it is always possible for an investigator to place healthier and more enthusiastic volunteers into the test group. If this happens, the better outcome achieved at the end might be merely due to the higher quality of the participant at the starting gate.

Besides equalizing group characteristics at the starting line, evaluation during the trial also helps demonstrate similarity. In the 1930s, the first major controlled study of the pertussis (whooping cough) vaccine was performed in Michigan. Vaccine was given to 1,815 children aged 8 months to 6 years. There were 2,397 controls. The active group was selected from all who presented themselves to the public health department requesting vaccination. The authors note this could have introduced selection bias. One might presume vaccine recipients were more likely to be from higher socioeconomic groups. Higher socioeconomic status is usually associated with fewer health problems. Interestingly, the study recorded two other infections, scarlet fever and measles, occurring in the pertussis vaccine and control groups. Scarlet fever struck 2.3% of subjects in the vaccine and control groups. Measles afflicted 8.8% and 8.5% of the vaccine and control groups, respectively. These intra-trial observations suggest the two groups were similar at the start and, more importantly, had the same infectious exposure and equivalent resistance to infection (Table 17.2).

There were 400 attacks of pertussis, 52 in the vaccine group and 348 in the controls. As a result, there were 2.3 annual attacks per 100 in the vaccine group and 15.1 attacks per year in the controls. Moreover, the attacks were more severe in the control group, indicating that when the vaccine did not prevent an attack, it ameliorated the disease.[13]

Table 17.2 Controlled Trial for Pertussis (Whooping Cough) Vaccine

Pertussis Vaccine Trial	Vaccine Group	Control Group
Number of subjects	1,815	2,397
Total pertussis attacks	52	348
Annual attacks per 100	2.3	15.1
Scarlet fever cases per 100	2.3	2.3
Measles cases per 100	8.8	8.5

Note: The groups were well matched as to infectious disease exposures and susceptibility to infections as demonstrated with nearly the same number of scarlet fever and measles cases. One does not need a statistical calculation to see the obvious difference between groups for the vaccine.

NATURAL HISTORY OF CIRRHOSIS

At the same time, the natural history of a disease should be understood. That is, if we do nothing, what happens over time to the patient with a particular disease? For example, what is the risk of primary cancer (i.e., not spread from another organ) developing in a patient with liver cirrhosis? Cirrhosis is a condition of a rock-hard liver with scar tissue replacing normal cells. Alcohol and viral infections can lead to cirrhosis. Before cirrhosis sets in, the liver is the only solid organ in the body that can regenerate. Cirrhosis prevents this regeneration. In a sense, cirrhosis converts a potentially immortal organ to a mortal organ. A mortal organ can be predicted. To answer our question, the cirrhotic liver has a cancer risk of 3% per year. Or, 1 in every 33 cirrhotics will develop primary liver cancer each year.[14]

Cirrhosis represents a stage of liver disease or a time place in evolution of damage. If one compares an agent that might prevent cancer in liver disease, they will need to ensure that patients in either the treatment or control group had cirrhosis properly diagnosed (inclusion criteria). They should also be free of cancer at entry into the study (exclusion criteria). Moreover, the control group for such a study should develop cancer in about 3 of 100 subjects every year. It is important to ensure the interventional group has not been declared better simply because the control arm behaved unexpectedly. For example, in a trial preventing liver cancer, the control group showed that 6 in every 100 patients developed cancer and in the intervention group 3 in every 100 subjects. The raw comparison might suggest the treatment was effective. However, the intervention likely accomplished nothing. The treated group behaved the same as the natural history of cancer in cirrhosis, while the controls had something odd happen. To sum up, a control group must be carefully selected, or it may become a misleading comparator. If not, the final conclusion may be a false-positive decision that the treatment was effective. False-positive means concluding an intervention works, when in reality it does not.

CONCLUSION

We have reviewed historical examples where solid scientific proof was obtained by comparing two groups. Disease definition is done through inclusion and exclusion criteria. The natural history must be well understood to ensure that the control group is not under- or overperforming.

Control groups help identify toxicity. If side effects are seen in individuals treated with a new treatment in an uncontrolled trial, the toxicity can be explained away. The desire for the new glittering treatment blinds us to the darkness within. How else can one explain the obvious toxicity missed with the gold treatment of tuberculosis in the seven years before Amberson's trial?

D. L. Sackett said it best, "Therapeutic reports with controls tend to have no enthusiasm, and reports with enthusiasm tend to have no controls."[15]

NOTES

1 *The Sign of Four*, Arthur Conon Doyle.

2 Roddis LH. *James Lind, Founder of Nautical Medicine*. Ann Arbor, MI: H. Schuman; 1950, pp. 48–50.

3 Ibid, p. 50.

4 Vitriol is an archaic name for metallic sulfate (iron or copper, etc.), and this was a mixture of sulfuric acid, alcohol, and spices.

5 A concoction of five herbs detailed by Lind in original passage.

6 Lind J. *A Treatise on the Scurvy: In Three Parts, Containing an Inquiry Into the Nature, Causes, and Cure, of that Disease, Together with a Critical and Chronological View of What Has Been Published on the Subject*. London: S. Crowder [and six others]; 1772, pp. 149–50.

7 Porter R. *The Greatest Benefit to Mankind: A Medical History of Humanity (Norton History of Science)*: WW Norton & Company; 1999, p. 295.

8 Gigerenzer G. *Calculated Risks: How to Know When Numbers Deceive You*. Simon & Schuster; 2015.

9 Diehl HS, Baker A, Cowan DW. Cold vaccines: An evaluation based on a controlled study. *Journal of the American Medical Association* 1938;111; pp. 1168–73.

10 Gabriel JM. The testing of sanocrysin: Science, profit, and innovation in clinical trial Design, 1926–31. *Journal of the History of Medicine and Allied Sciences* 2013;69; pp. 607–8.

11 Benedek TG. The history of gold therapy for tuberculosis. *Journal of the History of Medicine and Allied Sciences* 2004;59; pp. 76–82. DOI: 10.1093/jhmas/jrg042

12 Amberson Jr JB. A clinical trial of sanocrysin in pulmonary tuberculosis. *American Review of Tuberculosis* 1931;24; pp. 401–35.

13 Kendrick P, Eldering G. A study in active immunization against pertussis. With statistical analyses of the data by AJ Borowski. *American Journal of Hygiene* 1939;29; pp. 133–53.

14 D'Amico G, Garcia-Tsao G, Pagliaro L. Natural history and prognostic indicators of survival in cirrhosis: A systematic review of 118 studies. *Journal of Hepatology* 2006;44; pp. 217–31. DOI: 10.1016/j.jhep.2005.10.013

15 Sackett DL. Rules of evidence and clinical recommendations on the use of anti-thrombotic agents. *Chest* 1989;95; pp. 2S–4S.

18 Randomized Double-Blind Controlled Trials

Why care about bias? Why not make one group different from the other? Anyone can cheat.[1] The aim of research is to have others reproduce our results. Proof is strengthened when results are duplicated by others. Replication of data is what science is about. Contrary to the stereotype of serious scientists, there is a *Journal of Irreproducible Results* that publishes improbable investigations and unfounded findings. One strives to avoid being lampooned in this journal.

RANDOMIZATION

Despite defining the problem, the disease to be treated, and describing the people entering the trial, the investigator tends to place "better" (i.e., more responsive patients) in the test group. The process to overcome this bias is "randomization." Random in this context means the inability to predict the next number. That is, there is no predictable pattern. Research volunteers should be assigned by chance, not choice. The word random in this context does not mean "haphazard, careless, or indiscriminate."[2]

For example, if a trial were to plan 20 participants, 10 red (treatment) and 10 blue (control) slips of paper are placed in a hat and the slips stirred. The first slip of paper drawn out is placed into an envelope, sealed, and marked as "patient number one," etc. This would generate an unpredictable list of sealed envelopes. People not involved in the study should do this process. When the first patient has consented and passed his or her eligibility, the doctor can prescribe the test medicine or placebo as "subject number one's pills." The research pharmacist will open the envelope for subject number one and put the indicated pills into the research subject's bottle. The test pills and dummy pills should appear identical. This allows blinding for both the doctor and the patient (see the following section).

Some assert that a state of "equipoise" is necessary before randomization is palatable to patients. Equipoise refers to balance of interests. In this usage, researchers and subjects need to believe that both study arms possess potentially equal benefits. This is difficult to accomplish since too much prejudice exists in favor of the "new." The newly proposed treatment may not work at all, or it may have unexpected side effects. The placebo may even outperform the tested treatment. Thus, half of the patients are protected from what their doctors do not know about the treatment. It is this risk-limiting feature that makes concurrent controls ethical.

Most unproven drugs and herbal compounds when tested fail to work and often have significant side effects. The burden of proof is on the people introducing the drug. On the other hand, if the currently accepted treatment has firm scientific evidence supporting its use, then a new treatment for that condition can be tested against the conventional treatment instead of a placebo.

BLINDING A TRIAL

"Blinding" refers to the fact that neither the patients nor the doctors know which individuals belong to the intervention group and the control group. When only the patients are unaware, the term is "single-blind," and when both doctors and patients are uninformed, the term is "double-blind." One has to be careful not to use this "shoptalk" word (i.e., "blind") around patients, without defining it, since they may worry about visual blinding. In ophthalmological research, the terms "masked" or "doubly masked" are preferred!

If either party knows they are getting the "active" or "test" treatment, they may perform better on the basis of hope, or comply more closely with the treatment.

DOI: 10.1201/9781003324058-18

Blinding was first used to debunk bogus healers. Franz Mesmer (1734–1815) claimed to have found a new healing wave in medicine. Analogous to gravitation, he called this "animal magnetism." Because of the notoriety surrounding Mesmer's methods, King Louis XVI of France appointed a commission of inquiry composed of members of the Academy of Sciences. The American scientist and American plenipotentiary, Benjamin Franklin (1706–1790), headed the commission.

The first blindfold experiment was performed at Benjamin Franklin's house. A series of women who thought they could locate objects with the energy of mesmerism were physically blindfolded; then they were asked to locate where the mesmeric energy was leading them.

It may be observed that while the woman was permitted to see the operation, she placed her sensations precisely in the part towards which it was directed; that on the other hand, when she did not see the operation, she placed them at hazard, and in parts very distant from those which were the object of the magnetism. It was natural to conclude that these sensations, real or pretended, were determined by the imagination.[3]

Moving into the twentieth century, Rivers needs to be given credit for blinding of subjects in a controlled study when he lectured on his research on alcohol and fatigue in 1906:

One point of method has, I hope, been clearly established—that is, the absolute necessity that experiments with drugs on man should be carried out with adequate control, designed to exclude the influence of interest, sensory stimulation, and suggestion. Further, I have been able to show that this control is possible even in the case which seemed to me at first most hopeless— that of the administration of alcohol by the mouth. It is possible so completely to disguise the characteristic flavor that the subject of the experiment may be quite unaware whether he is taking alcohol or some inactive substance.[4]

Chalmers[5] presented definitive data about blinding trials in a classic article from 1983. His group reviewed 145 papers that dealt with the same diseases. Differences in case-fatality rates between control and treatment groups were obtained in 8.8% of blinded-randomization studies, 24.4% of unblinded-randomization studies, and 58% of the nonrandomized studies. Chalmers found these results were due to maldistribution of prognostic variables. Fifty-six percent of the variables favored treatment in the blinded-randomization group, and 77.6% and 81.4% favored the treatment in the unblinded-randomization and nonrandomized groups.

These and other data point to a general tendency to exaggerate the positive effects of a treatment by non-blinded assessors. This produces three scenarios. One, a small positive effect will become a large effect. Two, a treatment with no real effect seems to have a small positive effect. Three, and worse yet, a therapy with small harmful effects will appear to have a small beneficial effect.[6]

Blinding a trial is almost always necessary, but not absolutely. The author was the senior investigator and creator of a randomized controlled trial. The question was whether fluvastatin, a drug that lowers cholesterol, when added to interferon, would improve the cure rate of hepatitis C. The response to treatment, or evaluation point, was to reduce viral hepatitis C levels in the blood. In early studies of interferon treatment, a placebo had no effect on the levels of hepatitis C.[7] In other words, a patient cannot influence viral load levels with a placebo. After these studies, the Food and Drug Administration (FDA) no longer required a placebo group for hepatitis C trials. Instead, they encouraged a control group using standard therapy. Thus, in the author's trial, both patient and research staff could be aware of the group assignment since this knowledge would not influence the outcome. This is an "open-label" study. Nevertheless, two groups formed by randomization were still needed.[8]

The previous chapter discussed Sanocrysin. The patients involved did not know if they were receiving Sanocrysin or distilled water as an injection into the muscle. Side effects occurred only in the treatment group. Nausea, vomiting, and diarrhea occurred in 11/12 patients that took Sanocrysin, but none of the control group.[9] As a result, the patients likely deduced their treatment status. This latter outcome is called "unmasking" of the test assignment. If the trial had positive results for Sanocrysin, the masking could have led to skepticism of a false-positive outcome. In view of the damaging treatment results, the point was moot.

DOUBLE-BLIND TRIALS

Again, when both researchers and subjects do not know which group the patient is in, the protocol is double-blind in nature. Human curiosity being what it is, members of each group often attempt to guess their assignment. Success in subjects guessing their assignment during a trial leads to subjective but not objective improvement. Successful guessing bears no relationship to whether the patient finishes his or her participation in the trial.[10]

In any case, an investigator should avoid knowledge of patient assignment. A reliable method for this is to have a set of doctors who are not treating the patients make the final evaluation. For example, doctors not involved in the daily care of the study patient should evaluate the research X-rays.

Blinding both doctors and patients to the test treatment makes randomization palatable to both. "Randomization needs blind assessment. Blindness becomes the darkness enforcing randomization." The reverse is also true. "Blinding is only possible when randomization is employed."[11]

HISTORICAL OR REAL-TIME CONTROL?

Historical control groups are collections of subjects gathered from past clinical records. Chalmers's group compared the use of randomized controls and historical controls for clinical trials. For 6 common therapies, they collected 50 studies with randomized controls and 56 using historical controls. The treated groups in both the randomized trial (concurrent controls) and the current therapy using historical controls both had similar outcomes. The difference between the two types of trials is that historical controls fare far worse than studies using concurrent controls. This speaks to the bias of picking sicker patients to use as historical controls.[12] In other words, the tested therapy can appear to have better results if the historical group performs poorly.

THE BRITISH STREPTOMYCIN TRIAL FOR TUBERCULOSIS

The British trial of streptomycin for tuberculosis in 1947 is one of the first RCT trials ever performed.[13] The study randomized 107 patients—55 to the streptomycin test group and 52 used as controls. The trial included those with acute pulmonary tuberculosis. Patients were to be from 15 to 25 years of age (Table 18.1).

Physicians who did not know group assignment assessed the chest X-rays. Neither patients nor doctors knew their treatment assignment.

"A notable feature of this trial was the frank realization by all concerned of the fallibility of human judgment in general and of clinical and radiological judgment in particular. At all stages of the trial, then, precise criteria of diagnosis,

Table 18.1 RCT for Streptomycin against Tuberculosis in Young Adults

Radiological Assessment	Streptomycin Group		Control Group	
Improvement	38	69%	17	33%
No change	2	4%	3	6%
Deterioration	11	20%	18	34%
Deaths	**4**	**7%**	**14**	**27%**
Total	55	100%	52	100%

Note: The row in the table showing mortality is bold to illustrate the key conclusion of the trial.

progress, and cure were laid down, and all judgments on X-ray findings were made by two or more observers, independently of each other and unbiased by any knowledge of the nature of the treatment given to the patient whose physical status was being assessed. The principle of the elimination of personal bias is fundamental in all experiments, but it is of particular importance in clinical research. Thus, in the selection of patients for inclusion in either treated or control groups, the final decision was made purely on a chance basis. On the basis of these procedures, Reid[14] maintained that the effects of streptomycin on tuberculosis could be determined with confidence because 'we were reasonably sure that the rain of chance events had fallen equally upon the just and the unjust.'"[15,16]

The (now famous) statistician for the streptomycin study, Bradford Hill, advocated simple mathematics whenever possible for comparing two groups after a trial. If one focuses on the strongest and most unequivocal criterion of response (mortality), a clear reduction of deaths occurred in the streptomycin-treated group.

The use of the RCT format became increasingly common in the 1950s and early 1960s. Arguments persisted over the need for using the randomized controlled method versus clinical judgment—until a worldwide disaster hit.

THE THALIDOMIDE TRAGEDY

Public outcry against the drug thalidomide in the 1960s established the controlled clinical trial as indispensable. Without bothering to conduct controlled trials, thalidomide was introduced into West Germany by the Gronenthal company in 1958. It was advocated for anxiety and insomnia. Almost immediately, physicians began asking the company if thalidomide caused neuropathy (i.e., nerve damage). Company officials answered these inquiries in the negative and buried the correspondence.

Concurrently, an unusual type of birth defect was noted in Germany. But it was a long time before any association was made with thalidomide. Many scientists believed at the time that the placenta protected the fetus by not allowing drugs or toxins to pass from the mother into the developing fetus.

US law in 1960 allowed the distribution of thalidomide under the guise of "clinical trials." There were no FDA guidelines for clinical research at the time, and the company, Richardson-Merrell, introducing the drug into the United States, sought none. In early 1960, 1,200 US physicians kept nonstandardized research records and handed out pills to more than 20,000 patients. Of these, 207 were pregnant. There were no control patients.[17]

Richardson-Merrell then submitted a new drug application for thalidomide to the FDA in September 1960. They were confident of its approval within the 60 days allowed the FDA for review. At the time of submission for thalidomide, evidence that the drug actually worked in any condition was not required. The only data required was evidence supporting safety. The proof Richardson-Merrell provided was the lack of reported damage in 46 countries where thalidomide had already been approved. Or so they said. In reality, there were hundreds of cases of reported neuropathies. As many as 1 in 5 patients taking thalidomide for more than three months would begin to have prickly feelings in the feet with numbness, followed after a few days with numbness in the hands. The *British Medical Journal*, on December 31, 1961, was the first to publish nerve damage from thalidomide in four cases. Unfortunately, these nerve problems only partially resolved after stopping the thalidomide.[18]

Worse were the reports to the company that malformed babies were born if the mother took thalidomide in early pregnancy. The heartbreaking birth defects, called "phocomelia," consisted of limb-shortening malformations of the arms and legs. Gronenthal did its best to dispute and obfuscate the cause of these malformations, despite the deformities being unique in the history of medicine.[19]

Frances Kelsey, the FDA officer responsible for the review of the drug application, was a 48-year-old woman who had earned both a PhD in pharmacology and an MD from the University of Chicago. Despite intense pressure from executives at Richard-Merrell, she disapproved the application. None of the reports of nerve damage or birth defects were contained in the application for thalidomide approval in the United States. But even with the company hiding overseas reports of toxicity, Dr. Kelsey's response was that the company had failed to demonstrate safety of thalidomide in their four-volume application. During the review of the re-submitted application, Dr. Kelsey read the *British Medical Journal*'s *(BMJ)* report of nerve toxicity from thalidomide. When she asked the company's medical director if he knew about the report, the liaison sheepishly admitted the company knew of it, and he had no adequate reason for explaining why the *BMJ* report had not been included in the application.[20]

The application for approval was submitted six times, but the company never presented new data, just more testimonials. In the meantime, unequivocal evidence established that nerve damage and birth defects were related to thalidomide. Thalidomide was withdrawn worldwide. There were at least 11 cases of thalidomide-induced birth defects in the United States, but the exact number will never be known because the drug often caused fetal demise. The inadequate "research" records in the United States obscured final verification. Eleven cases in the United States, while tragic, are negligible compared to the estimated 10,000 birth defects worldwide from thalidomide.

That the FDA never approved the new drug application for thalidomide made Dr. Frances Kelsey a national hero. John F. Kennedy presented her with the President's Award for Distinguished Federal Civilian Service. Kelsey graced the cover of *Life Magazine*, the height of publicity at the time. The *Washington Post* headlined: "HEROINE OF FDA"

The public outcry in the United States led to the passage of the Kefauver-Harris Bill, known as the Drug Amendments of 1962. This law altered the basic character of drug research. It required (for the first time) proof of efficacy for new medicines. Second, labeling of drugs must disclose contraindications, precautions, and harmful side effects. Third, it strengthened the requirements for a new drug application. Finally, the law required the FDA to supervise the clinical testing of new drugs more closely. The result of this law would be the transformation of the FDA into the final arbiter of what constituted successful achievement in the realm of medical therapeutics.

What changed? As the law stated,

"Substantial evidence" [of drug efficacy] means evidence consisting of adequate and well-controlled investigations, including clinical investigations, by experts qualified by scientific training and experience to evaluate the effectiveness of the drug involved, on the basis of which it could fairly and responsibly be concluded by such experts that the drug will have the effect it purports or is represented to have under the conditions of use prescribed, recommended, or suggested in the labeling or proposed labeling thereof.[21]

With the passage of the 1962 law, the FDA set up specific guidelines. The conductor of the trial must submit a "reasonable protocol" based upon known facts. This plan had to contain data about the specific nature of the investigation.

With the advent of the clinical trial as a standard procedure, medical decision-making emerged as an issue of public policy. While drug regulatory agencies relied on the clinical judgment of physicians on their staff, the statistician's concerns took on increasing importance in assessing clinical trials. By the late 1960s, the double-blind, randomized, controlled methodology had become mandatory for FDA approval in the United States. Most large Western industrial democracies followed suit by the late 1970s.

RANDOMIZED TRIALS UNDER COMMUNISM?

Little is written on the subject, but randomized controlled trials were never performed in the Soviet Union or other communist countries. This seems to have sprung from their suspicion and banning of most statistical methods.

"The Russian word 'random variable' translates as 'accidental magnitude.' To the central planners and theoreticians, this was an insult. All industrial activity and social activity in the Soviet Union were planned according to the theories of Marx and Lenin. Nothing could occur by accident. Accidental magnitudes might describe things observed in capitalist economies—not in Russia. The applications of mathematical statistics were quickly stifled."[22-24]

No worthwhile new medicine was ever produced in the Soviet Union, nor has there been any other new meritorious medicine emerge from a communist country.[25]

Cuba is trying to emerge into the randomized controlled trial era. But it is beginning to appreciate the hurdles in doing so. To mention only a few, they are realizing the enormous funding needed to perform trials properly. All Cuban researchers point out the need to move from a paper chart system to information technology. Third, they must start by getting their research published in the world's medical journals, rather than Cuban publications. All global medical journals now require preregistration in international clinical registries before medical research involving human beings commences. This would require Cuban researchers to cease using their homegrown registration system. One wonders if the tightly controlled society can make the changes needed.[26]

RANDOMIZED TRIALS IN DEVELOPING COUNTRIES—BACKGROUND

Randomized trials in recent years have often been exported to developing countries. The reasons are a lower overhead cost and that certain diseases (e.g., parasitic infections) are much more common. A high prevalence of a disease allows a sufficient number of patients to be enrolled for a controlled trial. The numbers required for a study reflect the estimated potency of the test medicine. The number of subjects often needed is 200–400 or more. The incidence of parasitic infections in an entire Western country may be less than 10% of the latter numbers for a full year.

There are numerous advantages that accrue to the study population in any socioeconomic setting. Many of the author's research patients have expressed their satisfaction with the explanations they receive during a study about their illness. This information is presented in a detailed format prior to obtaining informed consent. Frequent follow-up visits provide the opportunity to discuss their illness and other medical problems. This allows them to more thoroughly understand their illness and achieve better care. The repetitive visits provide close observation, not otherwise available. In developing countries, this brings a standard of care simply not financially possible if the study was not performed. These benefits accrue, whether they receive the active treatment or placebo. Once the trial is over, if the test medicine has performed better than placebo and has no appreciable toxicity, the subjects in the placebo arm should be offered treatment with the now-proven study medicine. The study sponsor provides this aftercare at no cost. This is particularly true in the case of infectious disease. This latter requirement is considered an ethical duty of the backer.

In what is a relevant digression, the author needs to point out the vast difference between the abundant medical care available to those in the developed world and those in developing countries. This was made emotionally clear to the author after an invitation to attend the World Congress of Prison Health Care in Ottawa.[27]

It was of vital concern to the conference that international standards of health care for incarcerated individuals be developed. Setting such standards would help health-care workers stimulate politicians to provide greater resources to this vastly underfunded activity. For example, every prisoner should have access to psychiatric care. It seems intuitively obvious that this should be so. But a delegate from one underdeveloped country plaintively queried, "How can we possibly meet this standard when our country has only one psychiatrist for the entire nation?"

Or, what about prisoners having an adequate and nutritious diet available to them? Yet what if the general population in a particular country suffers from famine? In one case, prisoners in an African jail had to be released to forage for food with the needy local population, as both groups were going to starve otherwise.

The foregoing examples illustrate the social background of performing studies in developing countries. But the introduction of this section shows that many benefits can accrue to individuals and the community. Of course, such trials must be approved by the health-care administration and ethics boards of the local countries participating in research protocols.

RANDOMIZED CONTROLLED TRIALS IN DEVELOPING COUNTRIES

The challenges to performing randomized controlled trials in developing countries are numberless. The lack of funds and time for physicians is critical. Delay in approval and unskilled health authorities are also a barrier. Nurses are often what the West would call hospital orderlies. Inadequate infrastructure, such as computer networks, also poses a hurdle. Paradoxically, the need for reliable health-care evidence in developing countries is far greater. These nations need to prioritize the use of scarce resources.[28]

One problem not mentioned by reviewers presenting literature searches (of a sparse literature) at a distance is that in some countries real drugs delivered by relief agencies can be diverted to the black market.[29] Or the drugs may be switched with fake bottles looking identical to the original. The problem can be so severe that the makers of some proprietary drugs are forced to protect their brand name. To do so, local private investigators are hired to go incognito to see if the drug dispensed to the patient is actually present in the quantity and quality of the branded medication. By analogy, this diversion could easily happen with research subjects. In the final analysis, the doctor and researcher are unable to control what happens to the dispensed medicine when the patient leaves the building. Having them return daily for supervised pill taking is unrealistic since these areas have poor transportation options.

Our particular interest is in the debate over the use of the placebo in developing countries. Furor has arisen because the control or placebo arms have not always been the same as standard care in Western countries. The example often cited is the National Institutes of Health (NIH)–funded trial of using AZT in pregnant women infected with HIV disease to prevent maternal-fetal transmission of HIV. The protocol tested an oral AZT in women in the last month of pregnancy versus a placebo. The goal was to prevent the transmission of the HIV virus to the mother's newborn. Outcry arose because a placebo was chosen, rather than the standard of care used in Western countries. The standard of care at the time was an intensive regimen, called 076 protocol, which was started in early pregnancy. The regimen required compliance with a lengthy regime of oral AZT with repeated intravenous administration of AZT. Then, after childbirth, the mother had to avoid breastfeeding her child.

Unfortunately, the areas with the greatest burden of HIV disease are countries where women present late for prenatal care. Most women typically deliver their babies in settings not conducive to intravenous drug administration. Even if there were more hospitals, the few skilled health-care workers that do exist would be ill used to supervise large numbers of intravenous therapy for a research study. These African women also depend on breastfeeding to protect their babies from many diseases, only one of which is HIV infection. Moreover, the safety of AZT in countries where other diseases and malnutrition are higher than where the 076 protocol was used is unknown.[30]

> A placebo controlled study provides a faster answer with fewer subjects. ... [But] the most compelling reason to use a placebo-controlled study is that it provides definitive answers to questions about the safety and value of an intervention in the setting in which the study is performed, and these answers are the point of the research...[without this] it is impossible for a country to make a sound judgment about the appropriateness and financial feasibility of providing the intervention.[30]

The study of AZT versus placebo in late pregnancy was only funded, but not administered, by the NIH. The authors of the editorial defending the placebo effort received a letter from Edward Mbidde, chair of the AIDS research committee in Uganda:

> These are Ugandan studies conducted by Ugandan investigators on Ugandans. Due to lack of resources, we have been sponsored by organizations like yours. We are grateful that you have been able to do so. ... There is a mix-up of issues here which needs to be clarified. It is not NIH conducting the studies in Uganda, but Ugandans conducting their study on their people for the good of their people.[30]

And so it should be.

CONCLUSION

Even now, most countries do not have their own equivalent of the FDA for supervision of new (i.e., research) drug applications. Their regulatory agencies merely follow the guidance of the FDA on drug approval.

In sharp contrast, virtually all new medicines and proven medical treatments have been created by the industrial democracies of the West, with the United States leading the group. Japan has also contributed. Research methodology does help alleviate human suffering.

Why is the United States a leader? The author believes it has much to do with venture capital. That is, investors are freer in the United States to invest in drugs on the drawing table. It takes millions of dollars to support research of a new drug through the phase 1, 2, and 3 trials needed to present data to the FDA for a new drug application. These venture capitalists are at risk of losing it all if the drug fails to work as hoped. In fact, this is what usually happens. Yet, if the science and research methods are correct, a new drug can return a whirlwind to the investors. This is how risk and reward work. This freedom to invest and receive reward is stifled in many countries, particularly in those bent to strong socialism.

The author will not deny that the venture capital system and large pharmaceuticals have sometimes corrupted the process, but the FDA is a strong advocate for proper procedure. There is a delicate dance here for the benefit of humankind.[31]

Outperforming the placebo is now the ultimate proof in medicine. Controlled trials must be randomized. If there is a placebo effect for the disease studied, the study must also be double-blinded. One should take measures to rule out the "psychic effect" of a medicine on the patient. The physician-researcher must also avoid his or her unconscious bias. This unconscious bias can also be referred to as "honest subjectivity."[32]

Fair testing is needed with controlled trials to ensure that medicines help and do not harm.

NOTES

1 Indeed, there are famous examples of medical scientists actually faking their experimental data by making it up and fooling editors into getting it published. However, this is not the subject of this book.

2 Gehan EA, Lemak NA. *Statistics in Medical Research: Developments in Clinical Trials*. New York: Springer Science & Business Media; 2012, p. 92.

3 Franklin B. *Animal Magnetism: Report of Dr. Franklin and Other Commissioners, Charged by the King of France with the Examination of the Animal Magnetism as Practiced at Paris*. Philadelphia: H. Perkins; 1837.

4 Rivers WHR. *The Influence of Alcohol and Other Drugs on Fatigue: The Croonian Lectures Delivered at the Royal College of Physicians in 1906*: E. Arnold; 1908, p. 118.

5 While a gastrointestinal fellow at the University of Utah Medical Center (1986–1988), the author was privileged to meet with Thomas Chalmers in small group meetings. Warm and witty, Chalmers was well known for his ideas on promoting RCTs and scientific evidence. I recall him advocating that every patient treated in practice should be enrolled in an RCT. (See also Fein E. Dr. Thomas C. Chalmers, a President of Mt. Sinai, Dies at 78. *New York Times*, Dec. 29, 1995, p. 31.)

6 Robertson CT, Kesselheim AS. *Blinding as a Solution to Bias: Strengthening Biomedical Science, Forensic Science, and Law*. Cambridge, MA: Academic Press; 2016, pp. 64–7.

7 Davis GL, Balart LA, Schiff ER, et al., Treatment of chronic hepatitis C with recombinant interferon alfa. *New England Journal of Medicine* 1989;321; pp. 1501–6.

8 Bader T, Hughes LD, Fazili J, et al., A randomized controlled trial adding fluvastatin to peginterferon and ribavirin for naive genotype one hepatitis C patients. *Journal of Viral Hepatitis* 2013;20; pp. 622–7.

9 Amberson Jr JB. A clinical trial of Sanocrysin in pulmonary tuberculosis. *American Review of Tuberculosis* 1931;24; pp. 401–35.

10 Shapiro AK, Shapiro E. *The Powerful Placebo: From Ancient Priest to Modern Physician.* Baltimore: Johns Hopkins University Press; 1997, p. 202.

11 Kaptchuk, T. Intentional Ignorance: A History of Blind Assessment and Placebo Controls in Medicine. Bulletin of the History of Medicine, 72(3) (Fall 1998); pp. 389–433

12 Sacks H, Chalmers TC, Smith Jr H. Randomized versus historical controls for clinical trials. *American Journal of Medicine* 1982;72; p. 237.

13 Marshall G, Blacklock J, Cameron C, et al., Streptomycin treatment of pulmonary tuberculosis: a Medical Research Council investigation. *British Medical Journal* 1948;2; pp. 769–82.

14 A supervising physician from the Medical Research Council in Britain.

15 Matthews JR. *Quantification and the Quest for Medical Certainty.* Princeton, NJ: Princeton University Press; 1995; p. 132.

16 Last quote is an allusion to the biblical verse Matthew 5:4.

17 Stephens T, Brynner R. *Dark Remedy: The Impact of Thalidomide and Its Revival as a Vital Medicine.* New York: Basic Books; 2009, p. 43.

18 Florence AL. Is thalidomide to blame? *British Medical Journal* 1960;2; p. 1954.

19 Text will not illustrate these heartbreaking deformities. Readers can access images easily from an Internet search.

20 Stephens, p. 51.

21 Matthews, p. 132.

22 Salsburg D. *The Lady Tasting Tea: How Statistics Revolutionized Science in the Twentieth Century.* London: Macmillan; 2001, p. 148.

23 This is a corollary of Lysenko's bizarre science of "willing" the experimental result to happen. See the chapter, Soviet Science, in my book, *Wesleyans Help Women's Suffrage*, for the bizarre story of Trofim Lysenko.[24]

24 Bader T. *Wesleyans Help Women's Suffrage*. Revive Publishing/Amazon; 2018, pp. 283–6.

25 During the brief 79-year existence of the Soviet Union, it mocked Western society while also claiming to be the most scientific society in world history! Suppression of statistical evaluation may be one reason behind the ultimate failure of the Soviet Union. How can you use central planning to lead a society when you have no statistical data for direction? Recently, things have changed in the semi-communist areas of Asia.

26 Gorry, C. The ABCs of clinical trials in Cuba. *MEDICC Review* 2016;18 no. 3; pp. 9–14.

27 The author gave a talk on viral hepatitis in prisons.

28 Alemayehu C, Mitchell G, Nikles J. Barriers for conducting clinical trials in developing countries—A systematic review. *International Journal for Equity in Health* 2018 Dec;17(1); p. 37–48.

29 I discussed this with my college classmate, Gary Morsch, MD, who is the president emeritus and founder of the US private relief agency *Heart to Heart International*. He has been in over 175 countries. His agency has encountered all the problems discussed in this paragraph. *Heart to Heart* soon learned to have a predelivery agreement with the Ministry of Health of the country they were collaborating with. The agreement noted the inventory and manifest for the medicines and supplies to be given to each hospital. *Heart to Heart* volunteers then traveled with the medicines to each of the hospitals to oversee delivery. Further, the receiving hospital was required to keep records of lot numbers dispensed to the hospital pharmacy along with the final bottle number dispensed to the patient. These detailed records had to be of such quality as to pass audits of *Heart to Heart*. One tense encounter at an international airport provides an example. *Heart to Heart* arrived with their cargo jet to begin unloading medical supplies. A military unit drove up on the jet tarmac. The commander ordered the relief organization to hand over the pallets of donated medicines to his control. His military unit would see to it that they made it to the hospital. *Heart to Heart* representatives stoutly defended the predelivery agreement reached with the Ministry of Health. *Heart to Heart* staff and volunteers were prepared to repack the plane and return to the United States. A tense standoff with the armed troops then ensued for three hours. Finally, after communication with his government, the commander ordered the troops to stand down. The shipment would proceed under *Heart to Heart's* control directly to the receiving hospitals.

30 Varmus, Harold, David Satcher. Ethical complexities of conducting research in developing countries. *New England Journal of Medicine* 1997;337(14); 1003–5.

31 The author has sent numerous applications to the FDA and talked to their officers frequently. He has always found them reasonable and helpful in assisting a project but also strong in promoting proper regulation.

32 Robertson, p. 53.

19 Interpreting the Results of a Clinical Trial

So far, proof in medicine rests on the controlled trial and the ways to ensure that the two groups are as similar as possible. Now, we must determine if the treatment intervention was better than the control. Relax. This chapter will not require the reader to calculate numbers. Rather, we will approach them intuitively. We use numbers to navigate every day. What is your bank account? Why does it have the balance today that it does? Are we over the speed limit? Is the excess speed enough to attract the highway patrol?

We cannot substitute words for math. When friends say "more" or "less" or "greater," these are in fact calculations. Actual numbers provide far more precision. Regarding medicine, some might query what difference does it make? It can be the difference between life and death.

The simplest evaluation should be done, and this is often intuitive. Say we give a therapy for cancer in a test group and find 50 out of 100 people live for 5 years, compared to 10 out of 100 in the control group. One does not need complex statistics to determine the superior outcome in the test group.

Then, using the prior example, what if in the treated group there were 30 people that survived 5 years? At a glance, we would agree that the treatment produced better results than the control group. But then, like Abraham pleading for smaller numbers, would 15 survivors still be better than 10 survivors? What about 12 or 11?[1]

SIMPLIFIED PROBABILITY

The "probability value," shortened as "p-value," is an expression of chance, with a possible range from zero to one. What we want to know is, is the difference between the two groups interesting or not? What we compare between the two groups is their mean or average data set values.[2] In practical terms, the more similar the data are between the groups, the closer the p-value is to 1. The more the mean values are different (dissimilar), the numerical p-value declines toward zero.

The usual setting for an interesting study outcome is to determine if $p < .05$. This means the probability is less than 0.05, or 5%, or 1 in 20 of obtaining the observed results if the investigation was repeated. The usual way is to state that the comparison of the two groups is "statistically significant"; however, the latter phrase causes considerable confusion among neophytes. (The proper interpretation of the phrase "statistically significant" is discussed in the next section.)

What does the notation of $p < .05$ mean? An analogy can be made by flipping a coin. It is clear that if the coin is genuine, flipping it once gives a 0.5, 50%, or 1 in 2 chance of heads landing up. One can calculate the number of heads that can occur (from a binomial distribution) when a coin is flipped 20 times. If one counted 14 heads occurring when the coin is flipped 20 times, the probability value would be 0.037 (3.7% or 1 in 27); if 13 heads were counted, the p-value would be 0.074 (7.4% or 1 in 14). Thus, 14 heads observed out of 20 counted flips would represent $p < .05$, whereas 13 heads would not be $p < .05$.

WHAT DOES "STATISTICALLY SIGNIFICANT" MEAN?

Warning. The author refuses to use the phrase "rejecting the null hypothesis" to explain statistical significance. Using the term "null hypothesis" muddies the water. When "rejecting" is used to modify the null hypothesis, confusion reigns. How a double negative became ingrained into teaching a concept eludes the author. Hopefully, future thinkers can discard the double negative and simplify the explanation of the topic.

 DOI: 10.1201/9781003324058-19

In the meantime, when comparing the test group and control group, there are only two basic observations. The comparison of the means is not compelling, or the contrast is of interest.

When the p-value is greater than 0.05, then it is not interesting; when it is less than 0.05, then it is a curious result. It does not mean the results are absolutely different. Using 0.05, or 5%, or 1 in 20, as a line in the sand for probability cutoff is an arbitrary convention. In the beginning, it was a suggestion that has now become chiseled into the commandments of evidence-based medicine.

But this should not be so. We must remember the p-value is used to test hypotheses. In short, a lower p-value means there is less chance that the difference between the groups is just a fluke—an accidental result. But there are many things the p-value does not tell us. It does not tell us the magnitude of the effect, the strength of the evidence, or the probability the finding was the result of chance. Nor does it tell us if a larger dose of test medicine would have worked better.

Furthermore, it is necessary to consider the context of the RCT. If the groups were each a random sample of women over 50 years of age, then this statement on differences in proportion of survivors is only relevant to women over 50 years of age. Whether this statement can be generalized to women under 50 years of age or to men over 50 years of age is not part of this statement.

> A possible solution is to reconsider the nearly automatic use of a p-value of less than 0.05 as the critical point at which a difference is considered statistically significant. Perhaps well-designed and well-blinded RCTs with little chance for bias should be considered positive when alpha [i.e., p-value] is less than 0.10 or 0.20. This would increase the proportion of positive trials and save time and money. ... The decision about what significance level to accept should also consider other factors, including the prevalence of the disease, the medical and economic costs of the disease and of the therapy, and the best pretrial estimate of the likelihood that the new therapy represents an advance.[3]

A key concept the author is endeavoring to communicate is that there are two steps in evaluating a trial. There is statistical significance, and there is clinical significance.

Finally, clinical judgment is needed to evaluate the findings. The author can recall the discussion of one clinical trial at journal club where a new drug for constipation, designated as Drug A, was being tested in a double-blind trial against a placebo. When the data for Drug A was compared to the placebo group, the p-value was less than 0.05 and "statistically significant." However, only 30%, or 3 out of 10 patients, responded to Drug A. When the audience was asked if they, as an imagined investor behind the company testing the drug, should invest in further development of the medicine, most of the trainee audience thought the answer was yes since the study was "statistically significant."

My next question was, "Do you want your professional reputation to depend on a medicine that fails more than two-thirds of the time?"

This time, the answer was no.

Moreover, this treatment was for constipation, a non-life-threatening condition. There are many alternatives to treat constipation. Despite the trial result being "statistically significant," the company wisely elected not to further develop Drug A.

But we can substitute for Drug A in the prior example, Drug B, a compound with activity against a type of aggressive cancer that once it has spread from its primary organ, has no treatment options. In this case, if there is a p-value less than 0.05, we would take notice, even if only 30% of the test group responded. It would then matter how robust the clinical improvement was and how much longer the test group survived than the usual care group. Also, how much toxicity was suffered by the test group? Even though two out of three would fail to respond, patients might be willing to take this treatment if there are no other options.

Moreover, we would be willing to consider Drug B for further development against metastatic cancer if the p-value were 0.10 or 0.20. Perhaps, the enrollment of the test and control groups presented some anomalies. Or, if the chemical structure of Drug B was tweaked, it might become more efficacious and/or less toxic.

Thus, the interpretation of whether a trial is clinically significant depends on the setting of the medical problem. In context, statistical significance may not be important. Clinical judgment is needed to accept or reject the findings. One needs to ask, "Would the result make me change my clinical practice?" Like fire, the p-value is an excellent servant and a bad master.[4]

Bradford Hill reminded researchers that tests of (statistical) significance were being overdone in the medical literature. He felt there were innumerable situations where such tests were unnecessary and that "we weaken our capacity to interpret data and take reasonable decisions whatever the value of p."[5] Wisdom indeed.

CERTAINTY

There is never complete certainty about whether something works or not. The phrase "settled science" is an oxymoron. If, for example, we set a more demanding p-value of 0.01, and our trial results meet this more stringent demand, it will make it more likely others will replicate our trial (Figure 19.1). The lower cutoff will make it more likely that our study will be true-positive.[6] On the other hand, we have arbitrarily declared results of 0.02 to 0.05 as being negative. Thus, by definition, we have designated more studies as "false-negative."[7] We can have more certainty but at the price of excluding what may be helpful treatment.

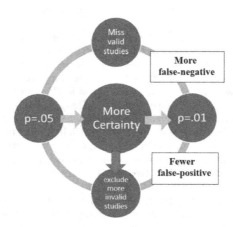

Figure 19.1 The effect of making criteria more stringent or specific. We can be more certain but at the expense of discarding studies that may be worthwhile. (Diagram created by author.)

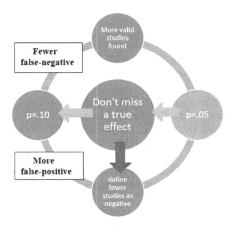

Figure 19.2 Making the criteria for p-value cutoff less stringent. We will want to do this if the disease has no other worthwhile treatment. Even so, a p-value = 0.10 would require further refined studies.

On the other hand, if we do not wish to miss any valid information, we can shift the p-value to be significant at less than 0.10 or 10% or 1 in 10 (Figure 19.2). This leads to fewer studies being defined as negative, and fewer will then be false-negative. On the other hand, adopting such a stance means more studies will be "false-positive."[8]

There is then no "correct" way to define the p-value for cutoff. It is often set at 0.05 or 5% or 1 in 20 probability for many disciplines. It is this p-value that is typically used to determine if the arithmetic means of the test group and control group are different in an interesting way (i.e., significantly different).

Then as we move right-to-left toward the left circle, we can turn the dial up toward p = 0.10. The left circle contains the expression "p = .10." However, setting the bar at p = .10 means that we may be accepting studies that have results that cannot be reproduced by others.

CONCLUSION

The basis of a controlled trial is to develop numerical data describing each arm of the controlled study. The data in each group will have a spread of numbers that can be understood as an average value or mean. It is this comparison of means that will determine if there is something intriguing going on. This contrast is expressed in a probability value. If the probability of these two datasets occurring by chance is less than 1 in 20, or a p-value less than 0.05, then in many situations this is declared "statistically significant," a potentially misleading descriptor. Statistical significance is a mathematical statement, not a clinical evaluation. It would be better to say the result is mathematically interesting. We then need to judge if the results are clinically relevant. If the trial found evidence for a new lifesaving drug, and the current treatment is miserable, one must not be a slave to the p-value < 0.05. One might pursue a treatment for further evaluation if the p-value was 0.10 or 0.20. Doing so would reduce the possibility of false-negative interpretation or missing valuable therapy. Just because the fire alarm is silent does not mean we should overlook the fire of potentially valuable therapy, effective new therapy that might be determined if the trial was designed with a better protocol.

NOTES

1 Biblical story. Genesis 18:16–33.

2 The comparison between groups also includes assessing the standard deviation (or standard error). Standard deviation is a number used to tell how much the measurements for a group are spread out from the group average. A low standard deviation value means most measurements are close (i.e., clustered) to the average. Practically speaking, this is a more reliable or reproducible result. In contrast, a high standard deviation means that most of the numbers are widely spread out. This is a less reliable outcome.

3 Sacks H, Chalmers TC, Smith Jr H. Randomized versus historical controls for clinical trials. *American Journal of Medicine* 1982;72; p. 237.

4 This is a paraphrase of Bradford Hill where he stated, "like fire, chi-square is an excellent servant and bad master" (see note 5 below).

5 Hill AB. The environment and disease: association or causation? 1965. *J R Soc Med*. 2015 Jan;108(1):32–7. https://doi.org/10.1177/0141076814562718

6 An effective way to remember "true-positive" is to compare this to a fire alarm ringing when there is a fire. This means the study is quite likely to be valid.

7 An effective way to remember "false-negative" is to recall that, the fire alarm is not ringing but there is a fire going on. Or, the study may have validity, but we are defining it as of no interest.

8 An effective way to remember "false-negative" is to recall that the fire alarm is ringing, but there is no fire. Or, the study may have validity, but we are defining it as of no interest.

20 The Gold Standard for Evidence-Based Medicine

By the early 1980s, the randomized controlled trial (RCT) became the "gold standard."[1] The classical gold standard was a system under which many countries fixed the value of their currencies in gold from the late nineteenth century until World War I. Now, the term "gold standard" is a phrase that indicates a high-quality target for comparison in any endeavor.

A RCT prevents human bias from sabotaging treatment interpretation.[2] There is no other way to test a new medical treatment. The new therapy need not be compared to a placebo but is often tested against the accepted standard treatment for the condition. One cannot use large pharmacy databases of patients to evaluate a new medicine, for the obvious reason that the new medicine will not be there.

The author estimates in his field of gastroenterology that at least half of our current treatments do not have controlled trial evidence. This is the "dark matter" of clinical medicine. While there are "treatments" for everything, the issue is—do they work? And as we have seen, most untested treatments are no better than placebo. Understanding this reality leads to therapeutic nihilism—"show me" the evidence before I accept it. In the meantime, we grope around in the dark matter and prescribe what other authorities advise.

In fairness, much of this dark matter contains treatments for diseases that are devilish to research. Randomizing groups for deep abdominal surgery is problematic. It is inadvisable to do a sham arm of no surgery for a ruptured aorta.

Many the vitamin deficiencies were discovered by omitting the vitamin under consideration in a bland-tasting formula fed to rats. These rats were kept in a cage for months to years with an exercise wheel. The controlled environment insured no other source of food ingestion. Since the lifespan of a laboratory rat is about two years, it does not take many months to observe diseases associated with deficiency or excess.

Chronic diseases, such as colon cancer or diverticulosis, may be due to improper nutrition. The onset of these diseases requires 20 years or more to observe. This is well beyond the research life span of investigators and the three-year financial grant cycle. Even the most agreeable research subject is unwilling to be given a bland diet, plus or minus the test substance, and remain in jail for 20 years running on an exercise wheel to nowhere. Human beings cannot control their diet outside confinement.[3]

Thus, how are these possible diet-related diseases, such as colon cancer, to be studied? Any diet intervention studies failing to show a difference in three to five years may be too short in duration. Or the subjects neglected to recall food ingestion, which interfered with the research question.[4] If the reader is incredulous, then in a more focused area, such as high blood pressure or diabetes, patients are notoriously unreliable in admitting their noncompliance with life-saving medicines. Noncompliance for hypertension and diabetes exceeds 50%![5,6]

CRITICISMS OF RCTs

To reiterate a common matter, patients are sometimes afraid to enroll in a controlled trial for fear of being randomized to the control arm—their prejudice is strong in favor of the new test medicine. They wonder if the trial is ethical. Why not just give the new test medicine to all comers? The reader has the answer by now. Ethics are not the focus of this book. But is it less ethical to prescribe untested medicines to suffering humans than to test these therapies?

We need to turn the question around. Odds are that a new test medicine will fail to show it improves the disease. Second, untested medicines actually have a

Judged beneficial, shown to be harmful
- Hormone therapy in women for heart disease
- High-dose oxygen therapy in neonates
- Antiarrhythmic drugs after myocardial infarction
- Fluoride treatment for osteoporosis
- Bed rest in twin pregnancy

Judged harmful, shown to be beneficial
- Beta blockers in heart failure
- Digoxin after myocardial infarction

Figure 20.1 Reversals in clinical judgment caused by results from RCTs.[7,8]

significant possibility of causing harm. And, worse, without prior comparative testing, we may not even appreciate the harm being caused (e.g., thalidomide).

A frequent question relates to the fact that a controlled trial examines only one dose of the test medicine versus placebo. What would happen if the dose was doubled throughout the study? Would there not be a better effect on the disease?

When failure occurs, the "more might be better" seems to be the reflex response. "What if" ruminations have resounded throughout history. Generals losing a battle wonder if more troops could have won. Defeated politicians wonder if more money might have succeeded. Maybe.

The problem in therapeutics is that there is often a fine line between helping and hurting. This may be best illustrated by the inverted "U"-shape diagram (i.e., "∩"). Many medications have this shape of response. Examples here would be alpha-interferon activity against hepatitis C. Increasing the dose augments the antiviral effect up to about 6 million units/day before the response plateaus. This plateau continues until 15 million units/day when one encounters a pro-viral effect. The author demonstrated the same phenomenon with a statin that has the greatest anti-hepatitis C effect with a small dose, but none at higher doses.[9] Thus, more is not always better.

Typically, the dose of greatest interest has been determined by a phase 1 study, whereby a few individuals (often less than 20) are monitored for the

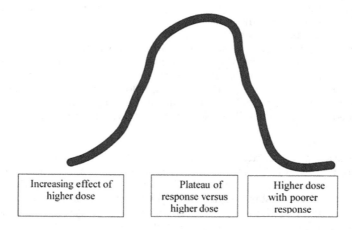

| Increasing effect of higher dose | Plateau of response versus higher dose | Higher dose with poorer response |

Figure 20.2 Dose-response can resemble an inverted "U" shape. With many medications, a higher dose leads to a poorer or lost response.

desired effect. Escalation of doses takes place, while also watching closely for side effects. If all goes well, then a phase 2 trial is performed. The two or three best doses from the phase 1 trial are then tested in 601/n100 volunteers to determine the optimal positive dose with the lowest side-effect profile. This optimal dose from the phase 2 trial is then chosen to be tested in a phase 3 trial. What we call an RCT is technically a phase 3 trial. This knowledge will help the neophyte, who wonders if a higher dose of an unsuccessful drug in an RCT would have worked.

Few people realize that virtually all controlled trials test only volunteers from age 18 to 75. Thus, for most therapeutics, the usefulness of a medication in pediatrics or geriatrics is extrapolated from data testing the 18- to 75-year-old age group. This inference, of course, may not be true.

The prime example here is the indication of using a proton pump inhibitor, such as omeprazole, for treatment of heartburn. There are no RCTs for patients with heartburn over age 75.[10] We just assume the efficacy and side effects are the same. But are they? We simply do not know.

The key issues in the group under age 18 are whether a valid consent to volunteer can truly be obtained. There are also fears that a side-effect experienced may lead to longer consequences. The hurdle for using research subjects over age 75 is more daunting. Death from all causes skyrockets. Mortality in the over age 75 group is 4%–5% per year. This means that if an investigator enrolls 300 patients over age 75 in a three-year study, as many as 12–15 patients could die from natural causes.

Alarms go off in the community and news media whenever a patient dies while enrolled in a research study. The alarm is due to the legitimate question of causation. Did the study drug cause the death? At its best, and most of the time, the death in the elderly participant has nothing to do with the study medication, as decided by an independent panel of experts. At worse, the investigators are tainted with an evil cloak. Still, in the duration of time required by the postmortem and independent panel to investigate, the season is stressful for both investigator and family.

The possibility of an annual 4%–5% mortality in a study of patients over age 75 has proved to be a major roadblock. Recently, the National Institutes of Health has attempted to encourage more studies in the elderly, with higher per patient grant funding and exploration of additional ways to encourage investigators to sally forth into this risky arena.

FINAL THOUGHTS

Our survey of proof in medicine has started from the long-standing humoral theory and its basis in authority. That is, it was true because someone who appeared to know something said it was so. Empirical testing began in the nineteenth century, and clinical judgment evaluated the results. In other words, one had to be a physician to assess efficacy. It was poorly understood that placebo effects could smokescreen real effects. In the twentieth century, controlled trials helped blow away the smoke of the placebo, but then we were left with two groups (i.e., control and test sets) with arithmetic data. Mathematics helps us decide if the difference between the average data in the two groups is of sufficient interest (i.e., statistically significant). In the end, clinical judgment is still needed to determine how relevant the interesting findings are. The RCT is not the only basis of truth for proving treatment in medicine, but it is the strongest and most durable.

It is worth reiterating that we must not become slaves to the p-value < 0.05. This is an arbitrary cutoff. Sometimes, the cutoff can be raised or lowered depending on how groundbreaking the treatment is or how certain we want proof that it is actually efficacious.

Much of the opportunity to record valuable data is wasted in the era of computers. If there is any doubt about the best treatment or dose, Thomas Chalmers was right to advocate that every treated patient in our clinics should be enrolled in a RCT. Patient information should be prospectively added, using research templates that can actually collect worthwhile data from ordinary clinical work. Perhaps clinicians willing to do so should have more time and salary to collect this data. We now grope around with retrospective attempts to gather uneven data from large databases.

We have criticized the old Greek humoral theory on many levels. Still, there is wisdom in the old Hippocratic aphorism—"first, do no harm."

We must remember there are only two types of treatment—proven and unproven. Proof is best established by the RCT.

NOTES

1 Jones DS, Podolsky SH. The history and fate of the gold standard. *Lancet* 2015;385; pp. 1502–3. DOI: 10.1016/S0140-6736(15)60742-5

2 This discussion assumes a high-quality RCT where patients are well matched, etc.

3 Who could stop the clandestine pizza run at midnight?

4 That is, the studies are false-negative.

5 Abegaz TM, Shehab A, Gebreyohannes EA, Bhagavathula AS, Elnour AA. Nonadherence to antihypertensive drugs: A systematic review and meta-analysis. *Medicine* 2017;96; pp. 1–9. DOI: 10.1097/MD.0000000000005641

6 Polonsky WH, Henry RR. Poor medication adherence in type 2 diabetes: recognizing the scope of the problem and its key contributors. Patient Preference and Adherence 2016;10; p. 1299–307. DOI: 10.2147/PPA.S106821

7 Ioannidis JPA. Contradicted and initially stronger effects in highly cited clinical research. *JAMA* 2005;294; pp. 218–28. DOI: 10.1001/jama.294.2.218

8 Rothwell PM. External validity of randomized controlled trials: "To whom do the results of this trial apply?" *Lancet* 2005;365; pp. 82–93. DOI: 10.1016/S0140-6736(04)17670-8

9 Bader T, Fazili J, Madhoun M, et al. Fluvastatin inhibits hepatitis C replication in humans. *Am J Gastroenterology* 2008;103; pp. 1383–9. DOI: 10.1111/j.1572-0241.2008.01876.x

10 Pubmed searched for heartburn, RCT, age greater than 75, proton pump inhibitor on April 9, 2019.

Index

Pages in *italics* refer to figures, **bold** refer to tables, and pages followed by 'n' refer to notes.